Path to a Healthy Mind & Body

*Connie Rogers Health Coach, Brain Health Coach, and
Published Author*

The content of this book is for general instruction only. Each person's physical, emotional, and spiritual condition is unique. The instruction in this book is not intended to replace or interrupt the reader's relationship with a physician or other professional. Please consult your doctor for matters pertaining to specific medical conditions.

Foreword

"Connie has a very well rounded and in-depth knowledge of health and wellness. She understands the complex integration of diet, physiology and well being along with the neuromuscular system. She is very passionate about teaching and supports you fully, while you take those "bite size steps" across the finish line."

"Finally her book encompasses what true health really means."

Michael Costello, Athlete, and Professional Contractor, Breckenridge CO.
www.summitcraftsmanhomesllc.com

Table of Contents

About the Author

From my earliest memories, I've always been a highly sensitive person. Born in an era when children were to be seen and not heard, I tried hard to make myself heard. Abuse was normal. I imagined I was dreaming and this scenario was not my life. Conversations in my head checked in often with my vital signs, "I have a family, I wasn't hungry, I was slapped around, mother had headaches and I wasn't supposed to talk about it." The term 'emotionally sterile' wasn't invented yet. Every day I thought about running away.

In school I found my creative flare was in socializing, team sports, and the arts.

In the 7th grade I already knew what my calling was: An aspiring artist in hair, makeup, and skin. At age 17 the Golden State called my name with a 6.7 earthquake in 1971. California was the land of opportunity and they don't have emotionally unstable people there, I thought.

The music that inspired me the most at that time was John Denver's "You Fill Up My Senses," Elvis Presley's version of "The Wonder of You!" and The Beatles® "A Hard Day's Night" album.

In California, I was able to make my dream come true, by becoming a Certified Cosmetologist. That same year (1977) I gave birth to my son.

I landed my first job as a skin care therapist in a day spa within a popular Recreation Center. That's where I met Greg, a hairdresser. I was the new kid on the block and was enamored with Greg, sponging up the tricks of the trade, watching every business move he made. Greg was never without clients. He treated them with the professional touch that only he was famous for, never rushing the client from the moment she sat in his chair. Women came from miles around just to have an appointment with Greg. After a while, I discovered his personal life was not on the same page as his business life. He sipped through life and women with a sense of humor, lots of parties, but never addressing his depression. Greg's depression and poor food habits continued for as long as I'd known him. One day he announced to all of us at the salon that he had found the woman he wanted to marry. We were all so happy for him. Three weeks after their wedding, Greg was dead. He died of colon cancer. What I noticed was Greg never took any of those precious moments, he so freely gave to all his clients, to give to himself.

As a California day-spa owner in the early 80s, and before it was common knowledge, I was already on the path of combining the foundations of healthy skin with my growing appetite for what we eat matters. Being an avid reader, I identified with and was drawn to a number of enlightening books by Caroline Myss. Her books titled *The Anatomy of the Spirit, The Creation of Health*, and *Why People Don't Heal & How They Can,* served to broaden my spectrum and passion about mind/ body health. Other additions to my library were: Tony Robbins: *Personal Power*®, Harriet Lerner: *The Dance of Anger,* Susan Jeffers: *Feel the Fear and Do It Anyway,* Paul Pitchford:

Healing With Whole Foods, Annemarie Colbin: *Food & Healing*, a relationship between food and health.

These authors shaped my life and filled my mind, body and spirit with the insight needed to continue my journey on 'healing from within'!

Like me, my sister was no stranger to emotionally unavailable people in her life. In 2000, after years of ill health she was diagnosed with ovarian cancer. She was originally given six months to live but continued to love and live ten years after her original diagnosis. In 2009 doctors suggested she have a cholecystectomy. Her lifestyle included several pharmaceuticals, mercury and other toxic exposures in her business as a dental hygienist. She suffered from anxiety, depression, and toxic relationships. I flew into NY and supported her with healthy ways to stay nourished, books to read to relieve stress, fear, and anger, and steps involved in avoiding stimulants. She in turn helped me on my journey to becoming a health coach. In 2003, I studied at the Institute for Integrative Nutrition™ in New York City.

Other academic studies that informed my work included Don Hansen from the Weimar Institute. His presentations concentrated around the importance of implementing a 'NEWSTART' Program® that included lifestyle, nutrition and fitness.

As a Mind/Body Coach, I love helping people all over the world via Skype and by phone.

An on-going challenge that people express at my workshops is their trouble with both weight and energy loss. The question often is, "How can this be fixed?"

My philosophy is eat real, be real, stress less, and make time for your personal health and wellness. My holistic approach encompasses learning what pulls the strings on metabolic and endocrine-related powers.

There are commonalities when exposed to toxins that create imbalances, factors when ignored over the years disrupt our 'life force,' which in turn can cut our life short.

****

Connie Rogers is a Certified Integrative Nutritional Holistic Health Coach, Brain Health Coach, Certified Cosmetologist, Skin Health Expert, Published Author, Reiki Master, Mother of 2, and Motivational Speaker. An expert in environmental toxins that disrupt our endocrine, metabolic, and skin health. Owner of bitesizepieces.net Join her Facebook Community here: https://www.facebook.com/bitesizepieces/

Special Acknowledgments:

I can never thank my family and friends enough for their help and support. Thank you to all those who supported and encouraged me through the last year.

Special thanks to the following for their dedication and support that helped make the creation of this book possible:

To My Sister Ginny Kirk, My Brother Joe and his wife Melissa, My Niece Karen Kirk, My Aunt Ruth Rossi, My wonderful friends Steve Williams and Don Parsons.

Thank you to Claude Fennema Professor Emeritus and Professional Photographer.

A big hug and thank you to Robin Quinn for her Editorial Input, guidance and Manuscript Evaluation Services. www.WritingAndEditing.biz

I had the opportunity to study under Connie May Fowler, an incredible book writing coach. Thank you www.ConnieMayFowler.com

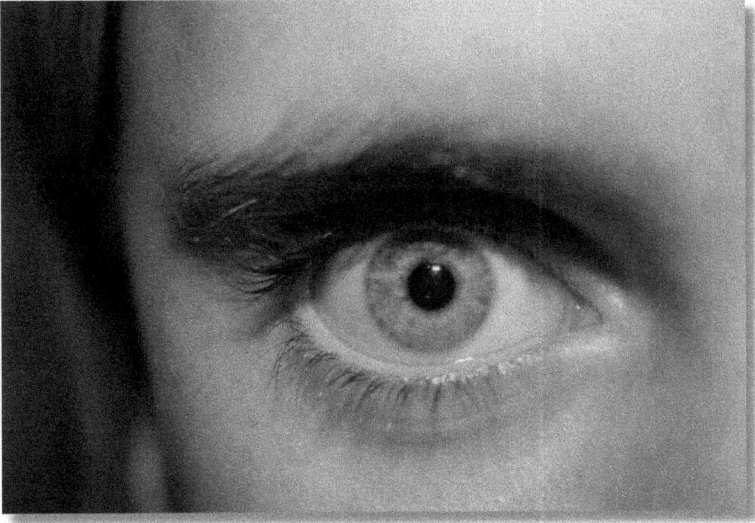

"Trust your instincts. Your mistakes might as well be your own, instead of someone else." Billy Wilder

Chapter I

Manipulated and Intoxicatedly Swayed

We've all had the devastating experience of losing friends and family members. Sometimes death comes totally unexpected while at other times it comes after long battles lost to preventative disorders. Saying good-bye to someone we care about is never an easy task. We often wish we had just one more moment, one more hug, one more hello.

I believe it's a myth that somehow a battle is lost when we die. My thoughts are that, in life and in death, it's not a WAR to be won. It's a journey of lessons, connections, and disconnection. A journey and destination that is entwined with opportunities that allow us to hold on or let go. A journey of touching hearts and souls. We touch each other often with our actions and words.

From an early age, we know intuitively what keeps us safe, what makes us feel good, and what does not. As adults, anxiety and depression step in and trick us into feeling powerless. What's missing is what's forgotten. We've forgotten that we have the ultimate power to make daily decisions that can shape our life. We've forgotten that holding onto misguided perceptions or a toxic belief system can keep us from moving forward toward our goals. We've forgotten that adding in elements of self-care and self-love is necessary for our survival. Bringing these elements to the surface of our existence today is the "Path to a Healthy Mind and Body."

There are choices we make on what we consume both physically and mentally. Harmful emotions or lack of proper nutrition in the mind and body can result in fractured cells, which become unable to do what is required to keep us healthy. Yet, if we let go of destructive habits, we create second chances for a new beginning.

Turning these pages forward can introduce you to a "plan." As you begin down this path, you will discover simple yet powerful steps with a plan to reduce the overload of stress, fake foods, depression, drugs, chemicals and pesticides that are all interconnected with poor health.

In this book, you can learn where and when false beliefs and misinformation squeeze their way into your subconscious programming. You will find that your gut and brain work in tandem, each influencing the other. You will become aware of what keeps you living the lifestyle of vitality — exercising or skiing into your 90s — or what keeps you sick, lethargic, and depressed in your 50s. In simple terms: *This book is a guide to living a long healthy life and that, simply put, is priceless!*

I love this great quote from Tony Robbins that asks: "When do people really start to live? [and the answer is] When they face death." I ask: "Why wait?" As you begin down this path to a healthy mind and body, ask yourself: *How can I live life and feel good each day?* This is instead of: *How many years is my life going to be defined by my condition?* It's no mystery that there are well-known dangers connected with drugs and alcohol. Less recognized is the impact of environmental toxins, fake foods and weight gain, which deplete our energy and cause inflammation in every one of the body's systems and organs. The truth is that helping our mind and body heal itself goes way beyond just managing symptoms.

Today there are still "Barriers" that prevent complementary and alternative therapies from healing us. Why is this? It's because, as Dr. Joseph Mercola has wisely stated, "while claiming public safety, there is a monopoly on health-care in the U.S."[1] There are various corporations that are designed to keep us safe. But they can also play a causative role in increasing our toxic load. Years ago, corporations advertised cigarettes were healthy for doctors, Santa Claus and the rest of us. Additionally, second-hand smoke from cigarettes was so sexy; it was good enough to blow in your partner's face after sex! Soda was advertised as a drink to serve to our children — the younger, the better. Advertising impacts the perception and attitude of a nation! Toxic perceptions and toxic attitudes can limit our decision-making abilities for a healthy life.

Remember, in recent years, ads tried to convince us that high fructose corn syrup, a "corn sugar" was natural and an equivalent to regular sugar?[2] Well it's far from natural.

This book carries with it a new way of thinking about what health really means. I think if people knew how they have been manipulated and intoxicatedly swayed with fake foods, fake science, and fake advertising, they would be totally enraged. It's time to create a path to a healthy mind and body, become empowered, and learn how to break through some of these barriers that are preventing your vibrant health.

---

[1] http://articles.mercola.com/sites/articles/archive/2011/12/30/rethinking-medical-associations-best-interests.aspx

[2] http://investigations.nbcnews.com/_news/2014/01/23/22406018-sugar-vs-corn-syrup-legal-battle-aims-to-establish-the-sweet-truth?lite

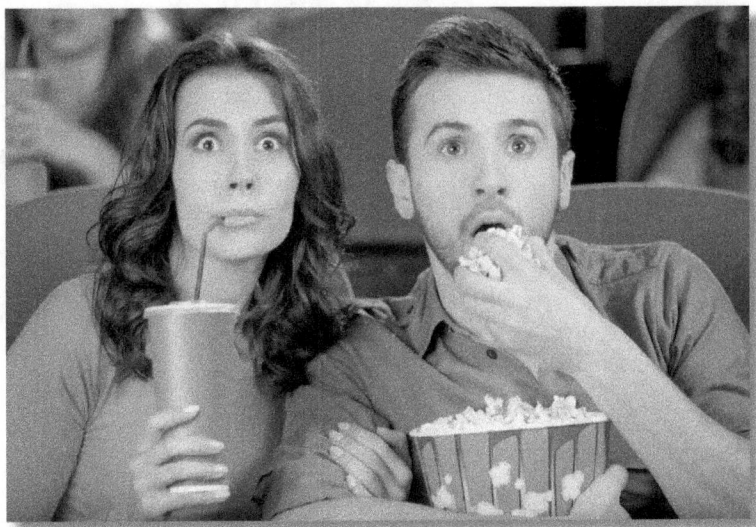

"There are about 280 million people who are walking around on earth who are addicted to sadness." Dr. Joe Rubino

Chapter 2

Stress Eating and Emotions

We are all EATING OUR FEELINGS in some way or another! I am no stranger to swallowing my tears and fears with sugar-coated chocolate chip cookies. As a child being abused and then given something sweet to eat was normal. Facts are when we eat under the influence of stressful emotions, we're not aware of how much we're eating, or what's eating us. The brain responds by slowing down circulation, minimizing any intelligent decision-making abilities.

Emotions such as depression, anger, fear, low self-esteem, feelings of abandonment lead to cravings. We want what we feel we're lacking, what someone else can't seem to give to us. There's a hole, a void, who's going to fill this empty space inside of us? We're consumed with feelings of instability, confusion, doubt and disappointments. We continue to eat thinking we can fill this void. And the stress continues.

TOXIC FOODS keep us from breaking the cycle of stress eating, by increasing the very stress we're trying to break free from. This is because toxic foods cause toxic moods. Inflammation takes hold and keeps the body in a craving cycle.

When we continue to eat in a stressed state, we can continue the cycle of stress through our entire nervous system, increasing fat and weight gain. This path can lead to diabetes, heart disease, cancer, and obesity.

Foods or Feelings? The body doesn't know what it's supposed to digest first.

The Gut-Brain Connection -
Laying the Foundation

Studies show emotional wellbeing RELIES on messages from the gut.[3] The gut is considered the second brain with the majority of serotonin produced in the gut than in the brain,[4] frequently affecting our emotional and physical health. (How we think and feel)

On any given day, emotions can control food intake, and food intake can control emotions. "Research on the enteric nervous system revealed many groundbreaking truths on how part of the nervous system in the stomach sends signals to the brain."[5] The unfriendly bacteria in our stomach are the controlling force that perpetuates inflammation in our mind and body.

"When we experience inflammation in our body, it is also in our brain." Dr. Daniel Amen

The connection between the brain and gut begins through the vagus nerve. The brain and the gut need each

---

[3] http://neurosciencenews.com/lymphatic-system-brain-neurobiology-2080/

[4] http://www.scientificamerican.com/article/gut-second-brain/

[5] http://www.ncbi.nlm.nih.gov/pubmed/24997031

other to survive. Therefore everything we eat, are exposed to, think, and feel, are aligned. "The gut microbiota is a therapeutic target for all brain-gut axis disorders." [6] These disorders include: Depression, Diabetes, Obesity, Alcohol abuse, Heart Disorders, IBS, OCD, Dementia and more. In fact, poor gut bacteria can be considered the greatest health threat of all time.

Thinking inside the box, medical professionals have significantly underestimated the importance of lifestyle for mental health.[7] Integrative Holistic practitioners like myself understand that to be healthy from within, the brain and the gut need open and healthy communication pathways.

This means less environmental toxic exposures and more high-quality foods to increase high-quality decision-making abilities in the gut and brain.

Leaky Gut Syndrome can occur when we don't pay attention to this gut/brain connection. An abundance of toxic foods, medications, chemicals, and stress keep our gut toxic and our brain sick. Undigested proteins and fats can 'leak' out of the intestine and into the bloodstream, where it sets off a toxic reaction. This is called Leaky Gut Syndrome. "When the intestinal lining is inflamed,…. there is often the mysterious and undiagnosed cause of infections within …other areas of the body."[8] This has a direct connection to all mood disorders.

---

[6] http://www.sciencedirect.com/science/article/pii/S0166432814004768

[7] http://www.apa.org/pubs/journals/releases/amp-66-7-579.pdf

[8] http://www.functionalmedicineuniversity.com/public/Leaky-Gut.cfm

Candida, <u>a fungal infection</u> from ingesting refined sugars, endocrine disrupting chemicals, or antibiotics, can be a precursor for Leaky Gut Syndrome. Candida disrupts hormones, microbes in our intestines, and our brain health. "When working properly the brain's circulatory system clears waste.[9] When not, waste remain. Leaky Gut Syndrome can keep the brain in a stressed environment.

> *When our gut environment changes,*
> *our brain changes.*

Have you ever been in a situation where it was so tough, you froze up? I have. When we act and react from toxic foods, exposures to chemicals, and stress, our perceptions can and will be altered.

Kathy's Perception

I met with Christine and her daughter Kathy in the parking lot of a restaurant. What I witnessed was a screaming out of control 15-year-old that for some reason couldn't be consoled. All her mother wanted was to hug her and make everything better. To the young girl, her mother's view was not her perception. The screaming went on for two hours,

---

[9] http://cen.acs.org/articles/90/i34/Brains-Circulatory-System-Clears-Waste.html

9

and I found it heart wrenching. Christine said, her daughter was experiencing severe PMS symptoms and didn't sleep well the night before. She blamed the antidepressants Kathy recently received from her doctor. I was interested in learning more and curious as to what exactly did Kathy have to eat that day to exasperate her symptoms? Was food, leaky gut or low serotonin levels to blame?

Serotonin is a neurotransmitter found in the brain and intestines. Serotonin does more than just boost moods. "It plays an important role in sleep, memory, aggression, cardiovascular activity, respiratory activity, regulating appetite, neuroendocrine function, but most important, perception!"[10] When given anti-depressants, these can alter our perception while the long-term use of antidepressants can deplete serotonin levels.

"Since 1988 the serotonin hype brought us several SSRI-Antidepressants." [11] *The Reaction:* "Drug-induced effects of antidepressants vary widely from sedation and cognitive impairment to agitation." Kathy was extremely agitated. As Kathy's story unfolded, she was also found to be allergic to gluten, which in turn plays a role in depression and leaky gut syndrome.

---

[10]http://www.medicalnewstoday.com/articles/232248.php

[11]http://www.ncbi.nlm.nih.gov/pubmed/10327841

When a Child Is Stressed

"Behavioral reactions to potentially stressful situations can alter the interpretation of stimuli. When a child experiences chronic stress it can influence his or her future health. The chain reaction can include cardiovascular disease, diabetes and more."[12]

Christine agreed to join my program so she could learn how to help her daughter balance foods, moods and hormones naturally. As a Certified Health Coach, together we took a path for wellness.

Do Corporations Perpetuate Depression?

Personally, I've had clients that were prescribed antidepressants and painkillers simultaneously. An ill-conceived perception is tied into a *belief system* that we somehow can't live without these pills. The cause and effect of this misinformed belief system can lead us down the road to cancer. We think pills offer us the opportunity to feel better now. Feeling better is at the top of our list at the moment. In reality, the body reacts by carrying the extra load of these pills, as they increase the symptoms of additional stress, liver toxicity, depression, fatigue, and disease.

- In today's world, Americans consume "eighty percent of the world's supply of painkillers."[13]

---

[12]http://www.ncbi.nlm.nih.gov/books/NBK43737/

[13] http://www.dailymail.co.uk/news/article-2142481/Americans-consume-80-percent-worlds-pain-pills-prescription-drug-abuse-epidemic-explodes.html

- Consequences from prescribed painkillers are actually killing more of us than street drugs, heroin and cocaine do in total. [14]
- Pharmaceuticals are known to contain sugar and unnecessary chemicals in the production of some medications. Sugar can increase depression.
- Thirty million people worldwide are being treated for depression and other mood disorders with antidepressants that can play a causative role to increase the very disorder they're trying to control. The World Health Organization states: there are 800,000 people that die each year from suicide around the world. In the U.S. suicide is the second leading cause of death between the ages of 10 to 24 according to the CDC.[15]
- There is more depression and illnesses in our world because of the years of exposure to *corporate chemicals* which in turn depletes our energy.

Are pills taking up real estate in your head? I had a neighbor commit suicide just last year. He was on antidepressants and just twenty-two years old. He felt his life was over because he couldn't financially support himself, and moved back in with his mother. Unfortunately suicide is so common, we are desensitized when we hear the news.

---

[14]http://www.healthfreedoms.org/death-by-big-pharma-painkillers-higher-than-heroin-and-cocaine-combined/

[15] http://www.cdc.gov/mmwr/preview/mmwrhtml/mm6408a1.htm

Jessie's Beliefs

Hitting rock bottom we can have good intentions to make changes, but if we're like most, everyday stuff can stand in the way of our belief system. Working overtime, the baby sitter's late and taking the dog to the vet can completely disrupt our day, stress levels and food choices.

Jessie describes an evening with her husband and children: "It's late, and pizza delivery is fast, cheap and easy. Everyone agrees. Finishing the day with ice cream after dinner, my husband and I turn off the TV and shuffle the kids to bed. Exhausted, I opt in for a few more hours on the computer, while I ice my neck pain. It's 2am and I find myself emotionally drained and bloated as I pop a pain killer. Another day without the time to exercise, I mumble."

We can't stop life. Even if our world is spinning out of control, it's human nature to want to embrace additional chaos. We fantasize about *having more time* to do more things that we want to do. Whether it be joining a gym or connecting with friends. We want to see results from losing a few pounds to healing from pain or depression, but only if we can find a path that takes the least resistance and the least amount of time. Unknowingly, we fall back on foods and ingest the medications that keep us disempowered.

Feeling lost and pondering a move toward eating healthier and implementing better lifestyle habits we dismiss that first bite size step. 'What's on our mind?' We forget that making small bite size changes and ultimately the results from these changes begin in the mind first.

If this sounds like you, time is not your enemy. *Beliefs are!* Beliefs can keep you thinking you need more time.

A Bite Size Step:
Find out what your beliefs are and what are just opinions.

Some Helpful Tips

'Beliefs' are critical to achieving your dreams. Creating a new reality can only come from new thinking. Ask yourself: "How can I be the best possible version of me today, even when things go wrong?" "What do I want?" "Who influences my beliefs?" If I've been carrying outdated beliefs around for 20-30 years or more, do they still serve me in my life today? And finally…is it possible to believe I have the power to change my beliefs and habits?

Old habits can lead to continued illnesses, brain fog and depleted energy. Or… new habits can lead to an abundance of energy, and better health with the ability to enjoy every day. What we say we want and what we do to achieve the goal can be two different things. But, it begins with beliefs.

Question antidepressants. There is a study, which suggests the term "antidepressant" be abandoned[16] because taking antidepressants do not add to the health of our brain.

_____

[16]http://www.ncbi.nlm.nih.gov/pmc/articles/PMC1472553/

> *"Until you value yourself, you won't value your time. Until you value your time, you will not do anything with it."*
> *M. Scott Peck*

Sue's Story

Sue is a signal mom. She's in my 'stress-less program' and sent me an email last week: "I didn't eat lunch, had a bad day at the office, and found myself caught in traffic and late for dinner again with the kids. It seems to be a daily occurrence that I arrive home hungry and agitated, and it shows. Maybe I'm not cut out to be domestic. Dinner was a disaster again. This is how my kids see me at the end of their day. How can I change this?"

Some Helpful Tips

My reply to Sue: Take a deep breath, smile and kiss the ones you love. They will forgive you. Look at what is possible for you to change that will work for all concerned. You can take the pressure off yourself by leaving work earlier or have a neighbor start dinner for you and the kids.

Check to see if you allow chaos to stand in the way of your relationships? Only when you get your principles in order can you fully show up, develop new habits, value your time and succeed in your goals.

Show up for self-care. Self-care encompasses every part of you, the 'whole' you, including your emotional side. Nagging thoughts and judgments about yourself can change your mood in seconds while at the same moment it changes metabolism and increases inflammation. Years of these habits and lack of self-care makes us all more vulnerable to depression and self-doubt, leaving our emotional and physical health and our family's health compromised. Kick self-doubt in the butt.

Find healthy ways to release stress. Work related stress could play a role in heart disease, thus affecting the immune system.[17] I invite you to view my 'Stress-Less Program' here.[18]

A Bite Size Step:
Ask yourself: How do I hold onto depressive thoughts and stress?

---

[17] http://eurheartj.oxfordjournals.org/content/early/2008/01/23/eurheartj.ehm584.abstract

[18] https://bitesizepieces.leadpages.co/stress-less-for-life-10/

Cognitive Dissonance and Willful Ignorance

Imagine a case of 'immediate gratification mindset,' (IGM) and how we've grown accustomed to it. We want computers, dinners and everything else in our world to run fast. We have the desire to move forward, but we find ourselves comfortable with the way things are. In this zone we are unhealthy. Now imagine some big corporation stepping in trying to fix it. The Department of Dietetics and Nutrition sees the problem from the eyes that we need additional medication to fix our disease and comments: "We're (people are) overfed, malnourished, sedentary, sunlight-deficient, sleep-deprived, and socially-isolated." They continue with:"Hopefully, this theoretical framework will aid in the understanding and treatment of depression." [19] (Treatment meaning additional medication.) But do we need another pill to fix our comfort zone?

An additional study examines the assumption that major depression is a specific illness; that is rapidly increasing, and that drugs may be the answer.[20] They claim depression is a mental illness and needs medical

intervention. Interestingly enough, Medical Research states LSD will be the new way to treat mental illness and addictions. [21] In reality, is LSD what we need?

---

[19] http://www.ncbi.nlm.nih.gov/pmc/articles/PMC3330161/

[20] http://www.ncbi.nlm.nih.gov/pubmed/18453728

[21] http://www.alternet.org/drugs/doctors-prescribe-lsd-anxiety

Depressed and out of sorts, we may feel that improving our condition is beyond our control. It's the culture that we surround ourselves with that teaches us to believe that we have no control. When in fact, the control is truly ours. It's the way we think, believe, eat and behave that allows us to take control or lose control of our internal and external environment.

Our Liver is Behaving Poorly

The Liver Reaction

Research tells us that toxic moods can be related to a toxic liver. We may have an unwanted behavior that hangs like a cloud overhead and for some reason we are *'stuck'* in the belief that this is where we must stay. This is what we know, and this place is *safe*.

When our day and nights seem to be filled with disappointments, we can find ourselves moody, and every time it seems to take a little longer shake it. *It's so much work being depressed.* Not only can food be a trigger to an out of sorts digestive system, the brain and liver together have a negative mood *reaction*. In fact, in Shakespeare's day, the liver was believed to be the seat of the emotions. [22]

Liver stress is when the liver cannot eliminate toxins properly. When this happens, all elimination systems can be compromised. If you are lethargic, toxic, moody and stressed, so is your liver. Have you witnessed crazy road rage or uncontrolled crying lately? What do you think may be the cause of this? Is it possible that more people are out

---

[22] http://drlwilson.com/Articles/LIVER.HTM

of control these days because they are extremely toxic? Yes, it is possible. The liver is our body's filtration system. How can the liver do what it's designed to do when we ignore all signals of distress?

Depression is a Disconnection Disorder

The body can disconnect when exposed to an abundance of medications. The number one drug in the U.S., is Abilify. This is a drug originally created for manic depression and bi-polar disorders. Now they advertise taking Abilify in addition to taking antidepressants. Six year olds are put on this drug for ADHD.[23] Abilify can cause irritability to regression. Side-effects include changing white cell count, brain function, and breathing. Last time I checked, brain function and breathing were important life functions.

Having a healthy digestive system is key to a healthy brain. Medications such as Zantac may increase the risk of cognitive impairment and depression. I've seen this drug given to babies. Antacids taken to fight indigestion actually diminish the enzymes needed to digest foods and nutrients critical to proper brain function.

Noteworthy: There are several cases where vaccines can be linked to depression, inflammation, and immunological challenges in the elderly.[24]

---

[23] http://www.circleofmoms.com/moms-kids-adhd/6-yr-old-son-with-adhd-put-on-ambilify-not-2-sure-how-to-feel-about-it-607049

[24] http://www.ncbi.nlm.nih.gov/pubmed/14557146 see also http://www.ncbi.nlm.nih.gov/pubmed/26348610

"A real decision is measured by the fact that you've taken a new action. If there's no action, you haven't truly decided." Tony Robbins

Decisions to be Well

What can steal your wellness? I will be the first to admit that there are certain circumstances that can drive us to a very low period in life. Thirty years ago I suffered a long and drawn out divorce, and the side-effect was severe inflammatory colitis. I held onto emotional pain and physical pain every day. Sleeping and eating was something I only thought about. Depressed, stressed, and overmedicated my gut was tired of the extra load. Drained and sick, my toxic body landed me in the hospital on numerous occasions. The side effect from the medication for colitis was kidney stones. I lost 30 pounds in thirty days and was severely anemic. To be a single mom and survive, I had to take a different path or die.

In my search for wellness, I dumped the medication, changed my eating habits and found ways to release my stress with exercise. Till this day, I have followed through with my decision to be well.

True healing, instead of a yearly detox routine, is within our reach but not often publicized. We can achieve better health and recover from a toxic mind and body when we change the habits involved that can perpetuate the cause.

A Bite Size Step:
Find out where you feel safe? What is your truth? Do you eat your feelings?

Some Helpful Tips

What if… we could make better lifestyle choices? It's easy to do when we discontinue life in the fast lane. Breaking this fast and convenient cycle requires a plan to be nourished and balanced in mind, body and spirit. It is possible to lessen our toxic burden and live the entire day well, with a conscience plan to do so. Happy moods tend to precede more health conscience choices.[25] *Take positive steps to eat your way toward happy.*

Foods that increase addictive type stress reactions in the brain include alcohol, wheat and white flour, caffeine, sugar, and foods that contain Excitotoxins. Excitotoxins include MSG, fluoride and aspartame. (more info on excitotoxins in chapter 5 and 6)

Besides interrupting digestion, eating these foods listed above can deplete our magnesium levels which can prevent the body from making serotonin. Serotonin keeps us happy, not caffeine and sugar.

So now we know, the gut influences and controls instincts, feelings, moods, health, and dis-ease.

---

[25]http://www.medicalnewstoday.com/releases/272873.php

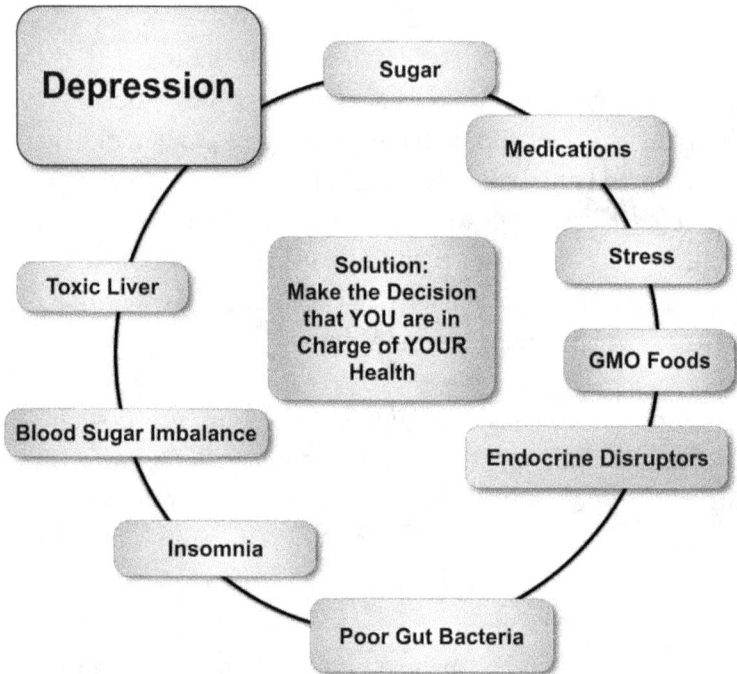

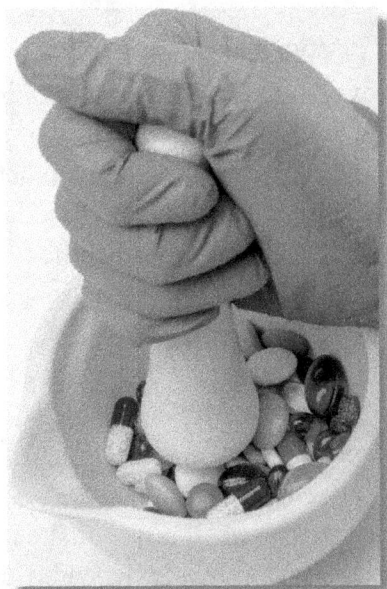

"We have a system based on maximizing profits rather than fostering good health." Andrew Weil

Chapter 3

A System That's Compromised

Chemicalized, Plasticized and Pesticides…
The industrial revolution and industrial farming brought with it dependencies', abuse, and overuse of toxic chemicals, pesticides, and plastics that are detrimental to the health of this great nation. The industrial processing and distribution system [26]is so harmful that the reactions from processed food choices can include cancers, depression and many other immune disorders.

Our world is surrounded by thousands of toxins, with only a few ever being tested for safety. This can mean our home and work environment and food security system has been hijacked. The *reactions*: can include dependencies on more than one pharmaceutical, just to make it through the day which increases the body's toxic load. Because of all these chemical toxins our core energy has become interrupted.

Adding to the general problem of toxicity in our food and environment is a fragmented health care system that is compromised by a pharmaceutical system maximizing profits over quality.

Often we've heard the phrase: "Follow the money trail." It can be found at the root of almost all global challenges. With focused online searches, we can discover very wealthy individuals and well-established Foundations put their money behind "drug-based research" resulting in a healthcare industry today where the masses are brainwashed to believe that pills are the answer. According

---

[26] http://www.ncbi.nlm.nih.gov/pmc/articles/PMC305362/

to the Thrive Movement Document, this alliance began in the early 1900's. [27]

Later on during World War II, Germany was instrumental in significant advances in drug research. Many of the large pharmaceutical companies today originated with companies from that war era that formed partnerships with these Foundations. After the war was over, some corporations were dismantled and later emerged as new corporations to form the food and drug industries interconnected with our U.S. banking system.[28]

Modern American Medicine Doesn't Treat Health and Health Care doesn't Include Care

As a nation, we are a drug system entwined into the very core of our food system. We have several new medications, and new smart and natural names for the same processed foods that cause illnesses and colon toxicities.

Television ads suggest, we ask our doctor for that magic pill. "Ask your doctor" is a catchy phrase for promoting prescription drugs. Believe it or not, this small money making marketing question has people racing to their doctor's office asking for the latest drugs, even if they're unnecessary.

Why is all this important? Because: toxic pills and toxic foods perpetuate the breakdown of the

---

[27] http://www.thrivemovement.com/drug-rx-money-making-killing

[28] http://www.sourcewatch.org/index.php?title=American_Medical_Association#cite_note-2

communication system between our mind and body. The end result ~ energy is lost, fear increases, and illness remains.

What if We Work Within Our Well-power?

Statistics tell us that most goals Americans set are about improving health. We assume these steps to health involve food, exercise, improved sleep, and less stress, with better-eating being number one.[29]

This could be one aspect of why we have so many New Year's Resolutions gone by the wayside. It's because these resolutions don't carry with them any real solutions. Why? Real solutions are found in *well-power!*

Well-power is the power within self in order to make change happen and continue for a lifetime. It's what makes YOU motivated.

The map to *well-power* solutions is in the guidance you receive from coaching. With a health coach in your corner, you are given the tools and the support you need to follow through and achieve the results you desire. Band-Aid approaches don't work~ results and success happen only when *well-power* is applied.

Research claims lack of willpower is why people give up their goals. But I believe wellness is so much more than willpower!

---

[29]http://positivepsychologynews.com/news/jeremy-mccarthy/2012060522562

If the American Dream includes health,
where is it hiding?

Wellbeing becomes insignificant when we allow disconnection between our mind and our body. Having the *mindset* to make wiser food choices is never as simple as it looks. Longtime toxic food habits and stress can stand in the way of our intention, leaving us open to depression and hopelessness. [30] Complacent, the body can no longer pay attention to its internal signal, to stop eating. The results: our weight loss efforts are hijacked. Recent studies show more than half of the U.S. is eating a poor diet with seventy-five percent being obese.[31] Poor emotional health and poor food choices weakens the immune system, leaving us less likely to make any new or longstanding healthy choices.

Some of us have had a love-hate relationship with our favorite moods and foods for 25 years or longer. Highly processed foods can act like drugs in the brain, causing *addiction.* This process can alter brain function, throwing self-control out the window.

So if we're talking about willpower....

Willpower doesn't stand a chance unless we address the true cause— corporate *conditioning, advertising and manipulation.* Somehow we unknowingly agreed to the poisoning from big food corporations, with an agenda to grab hold of our mind.

---

[30]-http://www.ncbi.nlm.nih.gov/pubmed/15363612

[31] http://www.washingtonpost.com/news/to-your-health/wp/2015/06/22/
americas-getting-even-fatter-startling-growth-in-obesity-over-past-20-years/

"Life begins at the end of your comfort zone." Neal Donald Walsch

Staying In Your Comfort Zone

You're sick and want to feel better, but your belief system stands in the way. You may have a **Yeah-But** way of thinking. I've found this to be part of the addiction process. You ask your friend why he's eating burgers, colas and fries every day. He claims: "**Yeah-But,** it was the only thing I could find to eat at the restaurant. **Yeah-But**, I was starving, I had no time for something else. Or …**Yeah-But,** it was yummy, I know I shouldn't have eaten it, but oh well." If you find yourself like a moth hitting the light on the downward spiral to disease, you may need to begin by breaking this cycle of addictive thinking.

If you're one that tells everyone "but I don't have time for…" Slow down, listen and think about what you just said. You said, "I don't have time for my health or my recovery, and I'd rather be sick and toxic. I accept the consequences of my daily addictions as normal for me. It's just the way it is and I'm not capable of changing my behaviors so, whatever…"

A Bite Size Step:
Ask yourself "Do I buy processed foods because it's convenient?"

Some Helpful Tips

Hidden toxic exposures can come from plastics. When plastics decompose they release toxic fumes and chemicals. PVC plastics can contain lead and phthalates that are toxins and found in our homes and our waterways.

Hidden toxic exposures can come from pesticides. Pesticides are in fact not designed to be safe to drink or eat. Yet they are found in our food supply.

Chemicals aren't designed to be digested. Yet we are exposed to toxic chemicals in our environment, water, drugs, and food supply. The body absorbs them and reacts by storing these toxins in our fat cells. Weight gain has more to do with the chemicals we ingest than willpower.

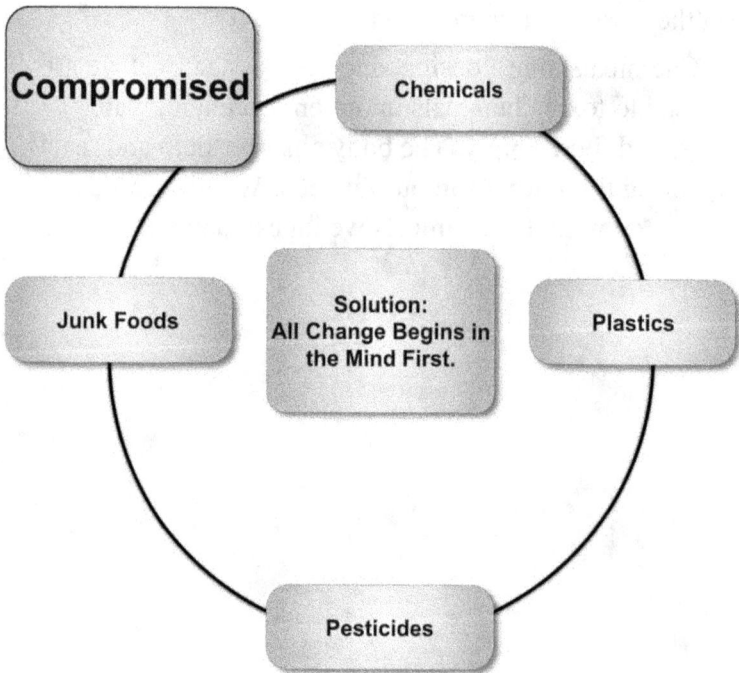

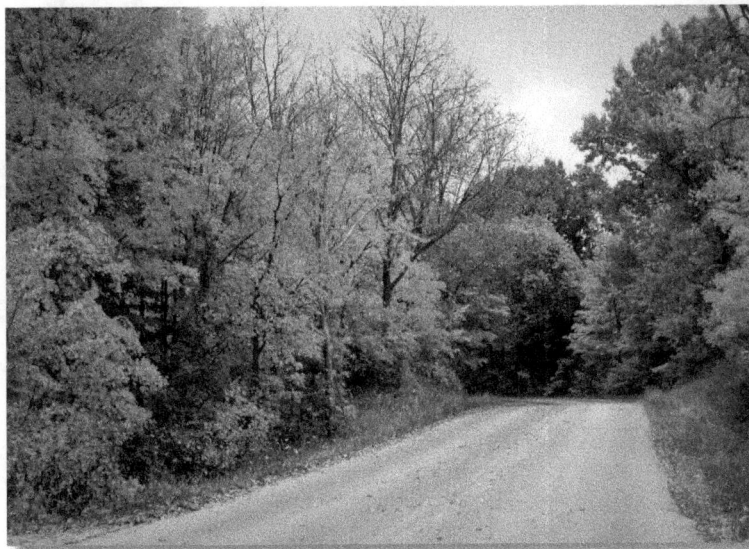

"Knowing is not enough, we must apply. Willing is not enough, we must do." Johan Wolfgang Goethe

Chapter 4

The Road Less Traveled
(Adapted from my blog at NaturalNews. [32])

---

[32] http://blogs.naturalnews.com/road-less-traveled/

Over the past century, millions and millions of people have been heading down a road. This road is now well trodden with years of habits that are deeply ingrained in our belief system as "normal." This road is not necessarily of our choosing but rather the results of billions spent in well-crafted advertisements by Food Giants and Big Pharma.

These giants give incentives and discounts for their products. Incentives to doctors to hand out samples of medications and discount coupons for you and I to save money on grocery store items. In a society that has also slowly grown into Global financial challenges as well, saving pennies becomes part of the driving force that impacts our decisions for health. On the path through these stores, we spend time traveling the aisles where the advertised foods and coupons discounts can be found. The Road Less Traveled is never a consideration.

> *Coupons for organic produce*
> *don't exist here in this matrix.*

At the end of each aisle is a tower of products "on sale" dumped in bins to be grabbed and added to the rest of our carts that are already overflowing with dead foods. Dangling off the sides of these carts, I see cases of diet sodas as if these are going to offset the junk foods.

The trip down the Road of Neglect continues with chips, dips, candy, popcorn, pasta, fried foods, donuts, cookies, all washed down with carafes of coffee and jugs of soda. Hours are spent in front of the TV with our favorite shows interlaced with beer, pizza and brainwashing advertisements. We don't remember the last time we did a push up.

If we're lucky, we have a friend who suggests that we might want to consider a few changes in our diet. Reality is that— the brainwashing from the bombardment of advertising, coupons and addictions stand in the way of our friend's suggestion. We enjoy these palatable foods we've been accustomed to eating. "It wouldn't be available if it was dangerous for my health," we say.

You may want to consider this...
In the delicate balance of the physical body we have approximately 50 trillion cells. Years of heading down this road "day in and day out" leads to a state of imbalance and breakdown of our biochemistry and bio- electricity.

At first we discover a small challenge. Maybe our blood pressure is a little off. The doctor is quick to write a script for a pill to address this symptom.

Together is it possible that all these are part of the problem, rather than the solution?

Looking For a Conscious Brain...

More people today feel something is missing in their lives, but they just can't seem get a handle on what it is. Addiction has set in. The brain is not fully focused.

Continued challenges show up with the addition of a new drug that has been added to our addiction of processed foods. Diabetes or some autoimmune disorder takes hold. After years of traveling down this Road of Daily Neglect, one challenge leads to the next. First our sex life begins to deteriorate.

The side-effects of the first drug is impacted by the side-effects of the second and the third along with contraindications of those drugs that are so often missed by the prescribing doctors. Then, fear sets in and we are "frozen" as we hear those words: "You have cancer and may only have weeks or months to live."

These words put fear in the hearts of all travelers on this road. I have witnessed the swift end of this "well worn road" with a stroke or heart attack. While for others, the road is a slow death from complications of medications and treatments.

> *So one might ask, "What if the people who were supposed to make us feel better were actually harming our health instead?"*

- According to a recent report the American Society for Nutrition (ASN) has "problematic ties" with "junk foods and beverage giants!"[33] This means they accept large sums of money from big corporations while they advise you and I what's best to eat. They publish the *American Journal of Clinical Nutrition.* What's really needed is neglected as we continue to stay a highly addicted and over medicated society.

- On their own site, the American Medical Association discusses the many possible avenues for conflicts of interest among their Board of Trustees.[34] Corporate profits have proven to be their number one concern.

- "Studies have found that doctors are the third leading cause of death in the U.S. [35] There are also medical errors and factors that kill around 250,000 a

---

[33] http://www.eatdrinkpolitics.com/wp-content/uploads/ASNReportFinal.pdf

[34]http://www.ama-assn.org/ama/pub/about-ama/our-people/board-trustees/conflict-interest-principles.page?

[35] http://www.ncbi.nlm.nih.gov/pubmed/17693227 see also http://www.ourcivilisation.com/medicine/usamed/deaths.htm

year.[36] And in addition to deaths and injuries, medical errors cost billions of dollars. A 2011 study put the figure at $17 billion a year.[37] To make matters worse, direct cancer costs are projected to rise from $104 billion to $173 billion in 2020 and beyond, with the highest costs incurred in the last year of life." [38]

Are you tired of this road that has been followed so blindly?

---

[36] http://www.jhsph.edu/research/centers-and-institutes/johns-hopkins-primary-care-policy-center/Publications_PDFs/A154.pdf

[37] http://www.sanders.senate.gov/newsroom/press-releases/medical-mistakes-are-3rd-leading-cause-of-death-in-us

[38] http://www.ncbi.nlm.nih.gov/pmc/articles/PMC3500487/

A Different Ending is Possible

The Road Less Traveled has proven to result in a different ending to this story. The price of purchasing organic foods over a lifetime along with the support from a health coach will never come close to the staggering cost of a road ending in cancer. The cancer journey is an incredibly expensive, destructive and painful one, for sure!
If you have the desire to take charge of your personal health, realize the Road Less Traveled is simply a matter of making a decision and being open to taking that first bite size step down a new path. The path to a healthy mind and body.

A Bite Size Step:
Follow your own road to personal health, joy, and happiness.

Some Helpful Tips

Most commercials continue to promote the road to neglect with their junk and processed foods. These include but are not limited to commercial yogurt, french fries, processed meats and cheese, canned soups, frozen dinners, sugary cereals,[39] crackers, salad dressings, energy drinks, processed energy bars, and bread. Be aware, some flours used in commercial bread-making can include potassium bromate that has been linked to cancer. When shopping at your favorite grocers, shop for real whole foods found in

---

[39] http://www.cspinet.org/new/201511091.html

the outside aisles of the store. Or, find an organic farmers market in your neighborhood.

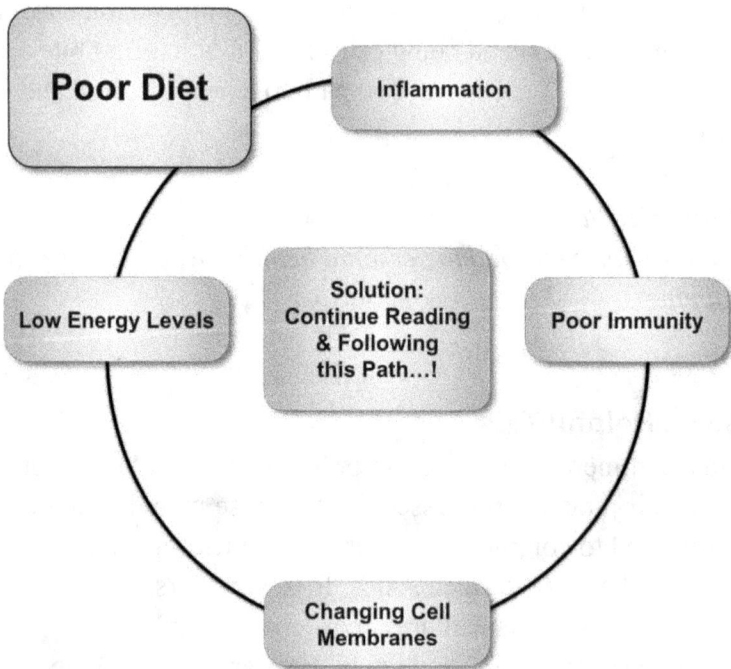

Poor Diet

Inflammation

Low Energy Levels

Solution:
Continue Reading
& Following
this Path…!

Poor Immunity

Changing Cell
Membranes

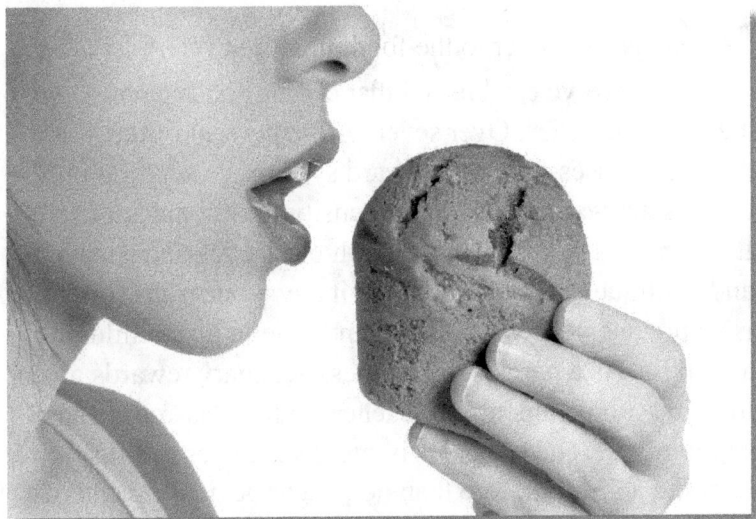

The Pleasure Traps

Chapter 5

When Habits Become Rewards

No one is a stranger to the food pleasure cycle.[40] In Chapter 2 we've established that certain foods have addictive qualities. Over seventy-five percent of the population uses food as a reward system. When food is used as a reward it has the propensity to become addictive. It begins at a very young age with our first birthday cake and continues into adulthood. Is it any wonder that obesity is so prevalent? In schools we find, one in three children are obese. As a parent, I've witnessed sugary rewards given to high school students by teachers in the classroom and at swim meets. The sad news is sugar sabotages a child's learning ability.[41] More than not, sugar begins and ends a child's day and is as addictive as cocaine. Sugary foods and drinks have been noted to cause and add to 'already depressive states.' Sugar also lowers Vitamin B12 levels in our body. When we are craving sugar for a reward it seems nothing else will do.

Adults use sugar as a reward after a hard days work in the form of alcohol. Yes, alcohol is sugar. The mentality is *it's 5 o'clock somewhere!* To find the courage to say no to a weekly cocktail hour, would mean to step outside the 'normal box.' Would we be accepted by our peers if we did?

Addiction to alcohol and drugs is an epidemic impacting more than eighty-five million Americans. Alcohol addiction can tax the heart considerably, causing high blood pressure and deterioration of the heart muscle.

---

[40] http://www.ncbi.nlm.nih.gov/pubmed/22487544

[41]http://www.dailymail.co.uk/health/article-2145141/Does-sugar-make-stupid-Study- suggests-sabotages-learning-memory.html

Alcohol affects digestion, lung and liver function.[42] In fact taking this one step further, alcohol adds to a toxic liver and gut which effect all other organs without exception. This can lead to insulin resistance and diabetes. In the U.S., one in three adults are diabetic.

Johnny's Story

Recommended by a friend, Johnny came to me severely depressed and hung-over. Alcohol was his pleasure trap. He had been told he had pre-diabetes and his limbs were visibly swollen. He lost his job, couldn't sleep, was stressed and didn't want to suffer and die like his dad did five years prior. Distressed from a budget-driven mindset, in the last 2 years he'd gained 59 pounds. Low energy and very poor elimination habits were what concerned him the most.

Johnny was sick and toxic and had a BIG reason to get well. (He didn't want to die the same way his father did.) I find in today's society, more of my clients are experiencing several illnesses at the same time, not knowing which one they want to address first. Johnny worked with me on incorporating new habits. Through all this Johnny heard what he felt was good news. There are many people that have been able to recover from alcoholism and depression. After 3 1/2 months, Johnny was on his way to feeling better. He continued with me for a year.

---

[42] www.medicalnewstoday.com/releases/55970.php

Is it possible for the body to heal itself? Yes. Johnny found life after alcohol addiction, and he was and is still committed to making necessary lifestyle changes.

"One needs to understand that they can have a potentially reversible condition and not a condition that is inevitably progressive."[43]

The Pleasurable Taste-Bud Syndrome

There are undeniable health risks involved with smoking and we've made great strides in combatting this deadly habit. Unfortunately, junk food is the new smoking habit. With an abundance of trans-fats, refined salt and sugar, our Standard American Diet is deadly. We won't let our children smoke, but we'll let them eat chips, bread, french fries and drink soda all day long. I see two-year-olds in the grocery store drinking an entire can! A pleasure mindset leads all of us into a 'toxic taste-bud syndrome'. This is where taste-buds control our mind— or— our mind is so addicted, it controls our taste buds. If taste-buds could talk they would say, "these flavors taste happy at this moment and that's all that matters." We may think we're experiencing pleasure, but we're far from it. The downside is continuing the cycle of depression, obesity and ill health. Once again, we lose the ability for any discerning decision-making.

Dr. Drew Ramsey, a psychiatrist, specializing in depression and anxiety, noticed very clear links between what we eat and the health of our brain. He said: "I think people intuitively know that, right? We all know how we eat affects how we feel." But do we really believe this?

---

[43] http://www.ncbi.nlm.nih.gov/pmc/articles/PMC3168743/

Food Stupor

There is also a "*drug-like effect*" in highly processed foods, which Corporate Giants use to keep us in this addiction stupor. The pleasure traps are usually caffeine,[44] burgers, sugar, salad dressings, ice-cream and the flavor enhancement substance known as MSG.

MSG is a man-made product designed to keep brains excited. We lose control while savoring these fake flavor enhancers in packaged foods and drinks, increasing the chemical overload that trigger our minds into craving more of them.

Some ice cream vendors 'soft serve treats' contain more artificial sweeteners, chemicals preservatives, corn syrup, and vegetable oils than actual milk products. These ingredients can have additive qualities.

We are sold a "false bill of goods" of fast and easy, store-packaged foods, with mouth-watering perfectly plated pictures of meals on the cover. These, we are told, are better, wiser and more economical. Many contain preservatives, chemicals, pesticides and a high refined sodium (salt) content.

Additionally our 'cheese addiction' can be blamed on a drug-like morphine effect (in the cheese,) and can be keeping us in an addictive stupor as well.[45]

---

[44]http://www.smithsonianmag.com/science-nature/this-is-how-your-brain-becomes-addicted-to-caffeine-26861037/?no-ist

[45] http://www.pcrm.org/health/diets/ffl/newsletter/breaking-the-cheese-addiction-step-3-cleansing-the

*Thus begins the hormonal disruption cycle toward
metabolic related disorders.*

TV is a Pleasure Trap

You feel comfortable eating by the TV for the last 35 years.
Sports is your thing, beer and pizza is your game. Why not?
Everybody does it! In the U.S. about 73% of men watch
football. Weight gain during football season is about 15 to
20 pounds for a season. If you sit by the TV longer than
one season, that can mean additional weight gain.

You may find it interesting to know that TV distraction can
disempower adults and children alike.

Children can also gain weight watching TV. They learn
very early on to emulate their parents. If there is no real
foods offered from Mother Nature's table. No problem.
Burgers, onion rings, fried shrimp, chicken wings with that
special sauce are the foods of choice, from freezer to
microwave to mouth. The sad news is, childhood pleasure
traps can lead to adult cancers. Are we going to fix this
deficit with supplements and enriched, fortified products? I
think not. The ramifications of a quick fix can continue to
compromise whole body health and lead us down the path
to pain, not pleasure.

Pleasure traps can also mean becoming a party animal. I
think we've all been there, myself included. I understand
it's fun having good friends over to enjoy good wine and

good food. What isn't pleasurable is vomiting from overindulging, after the party. Let's look at the reason why we think we need to totally overdo in order to experience pleasure. What makes us want to escape from being who we really are? With a little bit of digging, we may discover true friendships nourish us, for who we are underneath and inside out. When we are drowning with depression or addiction, we need help. That's when a coach is needed.

Bite Size Step:

Ask yourself: Does pleasure always mean indulging in additive substances, including junk foods, sugar, alcohol, or drugs? Find out what sucks you into wanting more of these. Remember, the goal is to nourish.

Rewarding Weight Loss

The are corporate rewards given when employees lose weight. Working with corporate employees I have heard many say: "If YOU want ME to lose weight, show me the money." Wow! Do you find a small problem with that statement? Does this mean corporations can count on sustainable changes from an employee, by giving bonuses for the most weight loss, no matter how it was achieved? Does it make a difference whether the weight loss was achieved by starvation or diet pills? Who wins when the employee eventually gains all the weight back, increasing the risk for lower immunity, more fat, and more doctor visits.

We might as well be talking about a slot-machine, when we say, "show me the money". Raising the stakes with weight loss, doesn't work unless there is commitment to oneself. We have to want to achieve true weight loss because we've made the decision to be healthy.

Without a frame of mind to "be-healthy" or "mindful" we might find ourselves with a limiting belief system, a fast, do it now, forget about the consequences later attitude.

Without a health coach employees can find comfort staying in that zone of ill health. This comfort zone may unconsciously keep them stuck, unable to step up or show up fully in their work environment.

Can preventing illness be less expensive than being sick? Yes, I would have to say, that prevention always cost less. However in health care, there seems to be a wide margin of beliefs preventing prevention. It could mean you believe you have no way out from hereditary ailments. It could mean you don't know where to begin or are afraid of the many unhealthy habits you've already formed. For corporations that believe health coaching programs <u>will make a difference</u> in the lives of their employees, and increase their bottom line, I invite you to connect with me here.[46]

A Bite Size Step:
What is your health worth? Success happens with a plan to move away from a non-committal attitude. It's the courage to see the bigger picture that will give you real pleasure to finally believe in yourself.

---

[46] https://bitesizepieces.leadpages.co/achieve-results-today/

Some Helpful Tips

Having a desk job doesn't have to mean bringing in cookies and donuts for everyone to eat. Try your hand at putting homemade lunches together. Purchase a water filtration system for the office. Weight loss isn't real unless you make real time for it. Benefits are: better elimination, more energy, and less stress.

Implementing a healthy lifestyle can feel good. You decide.

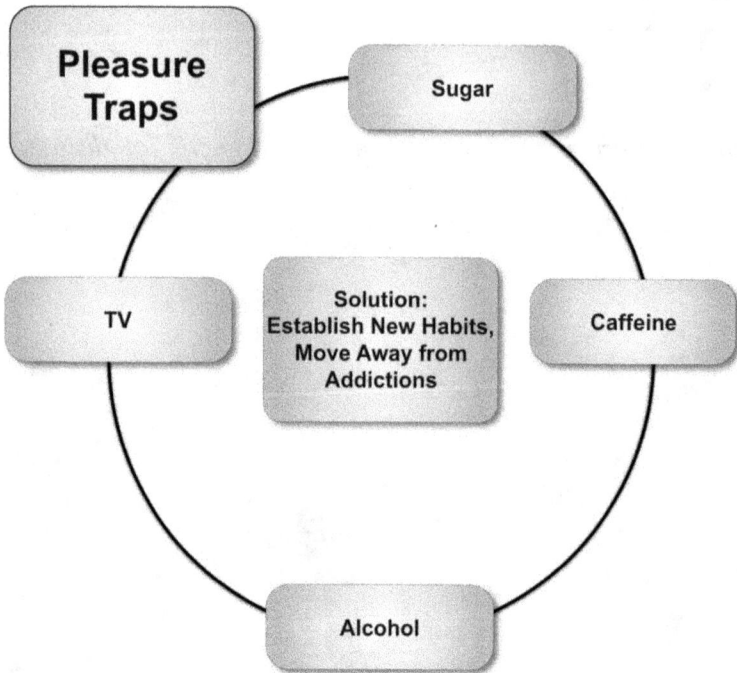

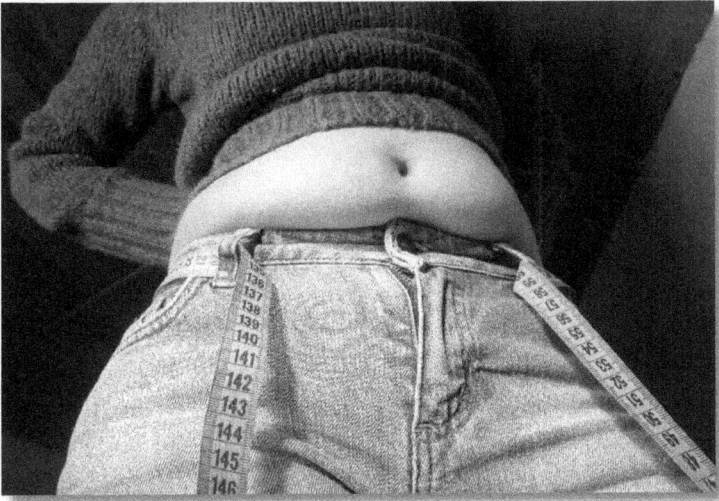

Statistics indicate some forty-five million Americans are dieting at any moment in time and thirty million a year is spent on weight loss products. If any of them were successful at keeping the weight off, we would all be thin.

Chapter 6

You're The Biggest Part of Me
(From my blog written for life coach radio networks[47])

---

47 http://www.lifecoachradionetworks.com/articles/2014/1/23/what-makes-true-weight-loss-different-from-weight-watchers-you-are-not-fat-you-are-toxic

Beyond specific nutrients and individual needs, getting nutrients from real foods - whole foods - nutritious foods - is really the only way to go for long-term health, controlling weight and obtaining quality of life.
Several theories say that to lose weight, all we need to do is increase our activity level and eat less. Theoretical equations sound so easy, don't they? But if losing weight really were this simple, why does the collective girth of the United States continue to grow? Most people get frustrated with dieting after a few weeks. Why? Because diets don't work. Ninety-eight percent of people give up and revert back to their old habits. Some say overweight or obese individuals are starving for whole foods and good nutrition. My findings are- this is only part of the journey.

The reason is that the old concept of: calories in, calories out, is not what's making us fat! Calories, a measure of energy, from a toxic food or a whole food, are never equal. The truth is, good fats are not making us fat either. Our 'Belly' actually needs good fats which balances moods and keeps us satiated. Our brain is about sixty percent fat. The right types of fats in our diet will impact our brain, weight, circulation, pain and inflammatory issues in a positive way.

However, there's another side to this puzzle. It's called: BIG corporations seem to be making the world fatter. Things we do on a daily basis, without thinking, can contribute to weight gain. The bottom line: The body has a hard time metabolizing chemicals!

Blast Belly Fat by
Reducing Hidden Triggers

Chemicals Keep Us Fat

Welcome to the new world order with exposures to over 80,000 chemicals that only a small percentage of which have ever been tested for toxicity.[48] There are new environmental chemical toxins, popping up yearly that we need to be concerned with.

- **Xenoestrogens**: We may unknowingly be ingesting xenoestrogens found in fake foods, commercial meat and dairy products, cosmetics, pesticides, household products and plastics. These add to weight gain and estrogen dominance. Xenobiotics can be found in drugs, environmental pollutants, skin care products, supplements and more. All add to unwanted weight gain.

- **Dyes** that have appeal: Titanium dioxide is used to make colors look brighter, is also a common ingredient in skin care products to make creams whiter and salad dressings for the same reason. The appeal is in the look! Titanium dioxide can be contaminated with lead, something we definitely don't want on our plate. Food

---

[48]http://www.psr.org/environment-and-health/environmental-health-policy-institute/responses/thousands-of-chemicals-on-the-market.html

51

dyes that are used on Easter eggs, in cookies, and in frozen drinks can contain unsuspecting chemicals and toxic aluminum byproducts.

• **Toxic Scents** are big business: Are you using dryer sheets, and spraying your favorite perfume or air-freshener in the air? Our sense of <u>smell</u> impacts obesity. There are avenues of environmental pollution that can be keeping us sick, fat, and toxic. Dr. Ruhullah Massoudi, lead author of the study from South Carolina State University Research, found that after just six hours of burn time, paraffin candles releases a significant amount of dangerous fumes such as alkenes and toluene, which are poisons.

• **Low-fat**: The low-fat fad diet promoted by the mainstream media is a misnomer in advertising. Why? Low-fat products can be loaded with sugar. Numerous long-term studies show that low-fat has never worked for weight loss.[49]

• **Medications**: Side-effects from medications can decrease any weight loss efforts. [50]

---

[49] http://jama.jamanetwork.com/article.aspx?articleid=202339

[50] http://www.lifecoachradionetworks.com/articles/2014/1/23/what-makes-true-weight-loss-different-from-weight-watchers-you-are-not-fat-you-are-toxic

- **Pesticides**: We are exposed to a variety of pesticides, chemical, bleach, and fluorides sprayed onto the produce we eat.

Our bodies are not separate parts designed to work by themselves. They are designed to work in harmony. Fat…"Adipose tissue is not simply an inert storage depot for lipids but is also an important endocrine organ that plays a key role in the integration of endocrine, metabolic, and inflammatory signals for the control of energy homeostasis."[51] Why is this important? Fat can lead to inflammation limiting the body's healing pathways.

In Floyd Chilton's book, *Inflammation Nation,* he said "Fat cells, themselves, produce the inflammatory messengers that cause inflammatory disease. The more fat cells you have and the bigger those cells are, the more inflammatory messengers you will produce, increasing …. an inflammatory disease."[52]

Are we Programmed to be Fat?

Even though fat loss is big business, there's a silent war going on against it. According to a food marketing report, the food and beverage industry spends [53]approximately $2

---

[51] http://care.diabetesjournals.org/content/26/8/2442.full

[52](Inflammation Nation, by Floyd Chilton, page 25)

[53] www.ftc.gov/os/2008/07/P064504foodmktingreport.pdf

billion per year marketing to children. The fast food industry spends more than $5 million every day marketing unhealthy foods to children.[54] One such ad claims it's OK to eat junk food while you're dieting.[55]

Some say obesity is caused on purpose in more poverty-stricken communities in our country and around the world. My thoughts are that it's a breakdown in our society that causes an obese mindset first. Maybe even complacency. Obesity is a global epidemic with many extremely toxic and natural solutions offered. Millions are made on weight loss products, liposuction, surgeries, and commercials offering misinformation and diets that can harm. Like a smoldering fire, we eat more and move less. Because of all these components we are programmed more than ever to be tired, sick and fat. Obesity is a man-made disease. Do you agree?

---

[54] http://www.preventioninstitute.org/focus-areas/supporting-healthy-food-a-activity/supporting-healthy-food-and-activity-environments-advocacy/get-involved-were-not-buying-it/735-were-not-buying-it-the-facts-on-junk-food-marketing-and-kids.html

[55] http://www.cnn.com/2015/11/12/health/dont-banish-junk-food/

In the U.S. we are ranked number one in childhood obesity

Belly Fat in Children

As parents I know we all want the best for our children. However lately I have seen more children under the age of thirteen, showing off their belly in ill-fitting summer clothing along with extremely poor posture. They appear depressed and seem expressionless. They avoid eye contact. Is this the new and accepted condition of our future America?

As a Health Coach, I've taught my 'Sugar Program' over 100 times to several high school classes. Doing so, I have witnessed first hand how children arrive for their first class in the early morning with donuts and soda. When children are so overweight they have poor self-esteem. Body-image and poor self-esteem are generally seen in conjunction with depression, and eating disorders. It's important to note if your child is obese, their body image is non-existent. The sad news is children can not learn on these non-food like substances. Countless studies and anecdotal observations confirm a clear link between the quality of food kids eat and their academic performance. In other words, a lifestyle of whole foods such as organic broccoli and peaches will likely get children better test scores than caffeinated drinks and pizza. And be honest – which foods do you see more often in the lunchroom?

The New England Journal of Medicine reported that if the childhood obesity trends continue, this will be the first generation of children that lives shorter lives than their parents. Why are we so concerned about test scores and ignoring our students life expectancy?

Diabetes is proliferating among our children, and half of all diabetic children are overweight. Remember when Type-II Diabetes was called 'adult onset diabetes'? Well, we can't call it that anymore, because kids have followed in our footsteps. And with that comes early heart disease and dementia.

According to The American Diabetes Association, about 208,000 Americans under age twenty are estimated to have diagnosed diabetes. When a person suffers from diabetes, adding in chemicals, colors and sugars can increase Advanced glycation end products (AGE) worsening oxidative stress and osteoporosis.[56]

---

[56] http://www.ncbi.nlm.nih.gov/pubmed/22023404

Some Helpful Tips

Stop waiting on weight! Grab your child's attention before depression along with obesity escalates into disease. You may want to rethink their sugar habit before you hand them over to Big Pharma. If antidepressants are recommended for your child, ask your doctor about additional weight gain.

Deceptive Ways We Are Tricked Into Fat

The mind and body are dependent on what we consume. There are imitation foods that are presented as real and there are toxic emotions around these foods that we haven't been able to shake since childhood. I've tasted them. The pastry shops, pizza parlors, and amusement parks are full of them.

When we feel bad, we naturally want more of that fake tasty food. It's an addiction that makes us feel even worse. We are paralyzed. Sounds a little crazy but it's true. Get enough chemicals, sugars, salts, flavor enhancers and artificial flavorings and we can be tricked into thinking or feeling it's what I love, or it keeps me happy. When, in fact, the opposite is true.

Some believe that if science is behind the making of junk foods, then it is one hundred percent safe to eat. My thoughts are this belief is the furthest from the truth. There is science behind the ingredients in junk foods that can make us crave more food and keep us sick. The ripple-effect has fat cells storing toxins.

Nine Examples of Fat Promoting Products:

1-*Chemical laden diet sugars* are advertised for weight loss. These actually program our body to want to eat more, not less. These endocrine disrupting chemicals disrupt leptin production and can interfere with weight loss. Aspartame is a known inducer of cancer because it can alter DNA. Anyone with lymphoma consuming aspartame, should be concerned. [57]

2-*Diet creamy protein drinks* that claim to be good for us are a waste of money for weight loss. The varieties include vanilla, strawberry, and chocolate. These contain chemicals and artificial flavors that fool our taste buds into believing they're the real thing. Personally I haven't seen any real foods on the ingredient list. Ingredients I do see are GMO corn syrup, maltodextrin, soy, synthetic vitamins, and milk protein concentrates (MPC) that are unregulated in the U.S.

3-*Diet powdered orange drinks* are promoted as yummy. They are engineered to taste just like 'orange juice.' These usually contains no orange juice at all. However, they do contain Aspartame and MSG.

4-*Liquid Sugar*. A term used for bottled, bagged, canned, or boxed juices. It is the largest source of sugar in the American diet.[58] Maybe fast and easy, but these keep us fat and these target our children.

---

[57]http://www.ncbi.nlm.nih.gov/pubmed/16507461

[58] http://www.sugarscience.org/sugar-sweetened-beverages/#.ViE3lLS29U5

5-*Packaged Dried Noodles* that appeal to people who want a fast and easy lunch. I see these noodles in the salon and spa industry. They are fast, easy, and filling. They are also toxic and contain ingredients that can increase our risk for metabolic syndrome.[59] (obesity, heart disease and diabetes)

6-*Spun Sugar* found at fairs and carnivals are a child's dream. These are usually made from refined GMO beet sugars, (beet sugar, a crop resistant to Monsanto's herbicide Roundup), chemical dyes-blue, red, yellow and artificial flavors.

7-*Movie Theater Popcorn* who can resist? These can contain hydrogenated oils, found in the fake butter flavor and yellow dyes. This popcorn, unless otherwise stated, can be compromised with GMO's.

8-*Weight Loss Frozen microwaved meals and desserts.* Found in most grocery stores. With heavy marketing, advertisers convince many that their foods are real. Almost all of these foods contain preservatives and additives that we don't really want in our body with many of the source ingredients being of the lowest quality and Genetically Modified.[60]

---

[59] http://www.ncbi.nlm.nih.gov/pubmed/24966409

[60] http://blog.fooducate.com/2011/05/20/weight-watchers-smart-ones-meals-not-that-smart/

9-*Liquid Fat*. Fats that are liquid at room temperature. They may include soybean oil, peanut oil and corn oil and are promoted as good oils. However, nutritionally speaking, these oils are some of the <u>most harmful</u> substances you can put into your body.[61] They can be rancid or made from GMO ingredients. As you can see, weight loss is big business combined with the industrial, pesticide and chemical big businesses that cause fat.

What do fat cells do?

• Fat cells store toxins.
• Fat cells increase lifetime exposure to estrogen.
• Fat promotes inflammation.
• Poor choices of fat compromises circulation increasing our risk for disease. Visceral fat is the fat around your middle located near the portal vein compromising circulation.[62] Visceral fat is biologically active and increases the risk for heart disease and decreases cognitive performance. After trans-fats, sugar is the reason we are fat.

That means the more sugar consumed can be deposited directly in our mid-section, the bulge.[63] In fact, a high sugar diet not only sets the stage for diabetes, it can play a

---

[61] http://www.marksdailyapple.com/healthy-oils/#axzz2r4VcXIJK

[62] http://www.health.harvard.edu/staying-healthy/abdominal-fat-and-what-to-do-about-it

[63] http://www.sugarscience.org/the-toxic-truth/#.VWpRWWC29U4

causative role for a fatty liver and obesity.[64] Why? Because insulin resistance and visceral fat decrease blood flow. Blood flow is important because the portal vein carries blood flow from the intestines to the liver.

Sugar interferes with hormones, energy loss, sleep patterns, calcium levels while increasing additional stress on all bodily functions. Sugar increases weight gain.

In Dr. Lustig book: *Fat Chance,* he teaches "excessive consumption of sugar is one of the primary causes of the obesity epidemic and metabolic disorders like diabetes, as well as of cardiovascular disease."

According to The American Heart Association there are 180,000 deaths a year from sugary drinks.[65]

What Else Can Keep Us Fat?

1-Frequent antibiotic use or choosing foods with Antibiotics can wreak havoc on our hormonal balance, causing inflammation and increasing our bottom line. Fat!

2-MSG, an excitotoxin, can be lurking in your pantry and freezer posing as salt. We can never lose weight on MSG because it's designed to make us eat more of it. If potato chips are in your pantry, check for this ingredient.

3-Lack of sleep can cause weight gain.

------

[64]http://link.springer.com/article/10.1007/s11892-012-0259-6

[65]http://newsroom.heart.org/news/180-000-deaths-worldwide-may-be-associated-with-sugary-soft-drinks?preview=5d39

4-Poor gut bacteria can cause weight gain. (See chapter 2)

5-Chronic intake of farmed fatty fish contributes to insulin resistance and obesity. These negative effects are found in the presence of <u>persistent organic pollutants</u> (POPs) inside farmed fatty fish. So it is safe to say eating farmed fish and suffering from obesity can increase the risk of fatty liver disease.

6-Hormonal Disruption. When hormones are disrupted there is little chance for permanent weight loss. Unbalanced hormones are connected to energy loss. Growth hormones in dairy products, not only disrupt hormones, they have been linked to cancer.[66]

Some Helpful Tips

Metabolism is all about energy. Whole foods from Mother Natures Table is eating for energy. Feeding your body and brain also includes scheduling some time for exercise. It's about a healthy mindset and knowing the interrelationship we have with food, toxins, lack of movement and disease.

Noteworthy: Look, taste, smell and chew your food at every meal. Avoid the 'shovel-effect' at the end of your fork. Food can be our medicine or our poison. It's simply a matter of daily choices.

---

[66] Cramer DW, Harlow BL, Willet WC. Galactose consumption and metabolism in relation to the risk of ovarian cancer. Lancet 1989;2:66-71. see also <u>http://ajcn.nutrition.org/content/80/5/1353.full</u>

Foods to Eat to Remove Belly Fat

Avoid gluten and eat mung beans. Sprouted mung beans are a great source of protein and fiber and considered a superfood.

Ditch the refined sugar and eat blueberries.

Spinach is a belly fat fighter and a must have at least two times a day!

An abundance of caffeine in your day can lead to insulin resistance. Caffeine can also add to sugar cravings. Instead, eat organic apples in the morning. Surprisingly, these can help you wake up without reaching for that hot cup of coffee and they help reduce belly fat.

Don't be tricked into eating yogurt. Store bought yogurts can contain unwanted sugars and are a pasteurized dead food product. Several options include making your own cashew-nut or almond yogurt.

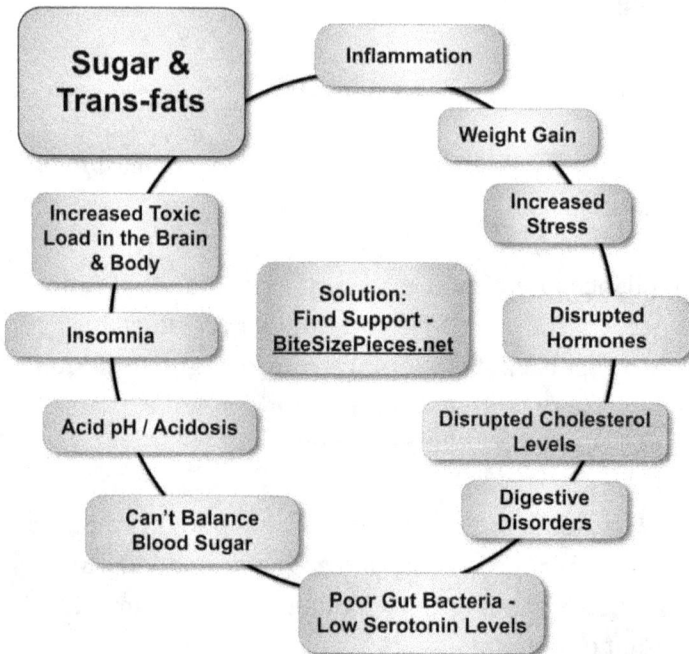

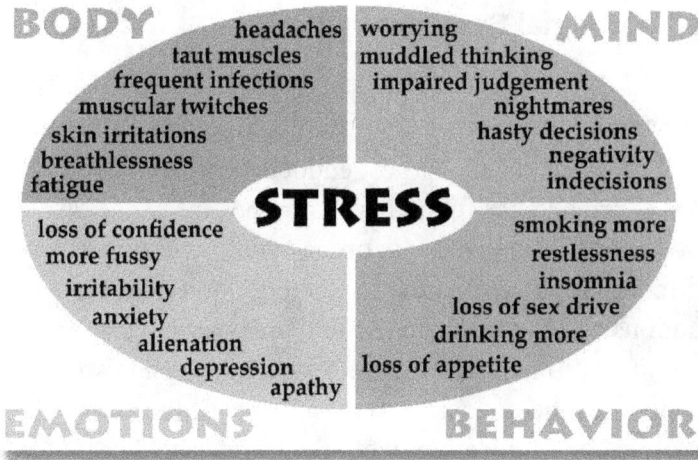

BODY		MIND
headaches	worrying	
taut muscles	muddled thinking	
frequent infections	impaired judgement	
muscular twitches		nightmares
skin irritations		hasty decisions
breathlessness		negativity
fatigue		indecisions

STRESS

loss of confidence	smoking more
more fussy	restlessness
irritability	insomnia
anxiety	loss of sex drive
alienation	drinking more
depression	loss of appetite
apathy	

EMOTIONS **BEHAVIOR**

"The question is not what we look at, but what we see."
Henry David Thoreau

Chapter 7

Endocrine Disruption

Our Hormonal System

The endocrine system is our hormonal system. The stomach is seen as the largest endocrine organ in the body.[67] Science has found that hormones influence all systems of the human body, organs and our brain. Hormones regulate metabolism, energy production, emotions and more. The brain and the body have a direct communication system via the endocrine mechanisms.[68]

Because the endocrine system is one of the most sensitive communication networks, endocrine disruption can keep us fat, sick and depressed. Endocrine Disruptors are chemicals, foods and toxins that mimic natural hormones, causing overproduction or underproduction of hormones. They are injurious to our well being, our environment and our water ways."[69]

Our endocrine system regulates metabolic rate, and endocrine disruptors- disrupt metabolism. So we can safely say that Endocrine Disruptors are the catalyst to metabolic syndrome. No one wants to age faster than normal or experience hormonal imbalances that can lead to unwanted weight gain, low energy, premature aging and auto-immune disorders. But in reality we seem to do it every day. Obesity, Depression, Heart Disease, Diabetes, and Cancer risk increase with endocrine disrupting chemicals.

---

[67] http://www.vivo.colostate.edu/hbooks/pathphys/digestion/basics/gi_endocrine.html.

[68] http://physrev.physiology.org/content/87/3/873

[69] http://www.psr.org/environment-and-health/environmental-health-policy-institute/responses/thousands-of-chemicals-on-the-market.html

According to Dr. Bruce Blumberg at the University of California in Irvine, "Commonly known 'endocrine-disrupting' chemicals include PCBs, DDT, dioxins, pesticides, and many plasticizers, like BPA."

Some Helpful Tips

Reach out and connect with me on what you can do to avoid endocrine disruption. Remember, a poor diet of processed foods and chemicals are continually disrupting our hormones.

Side-Effects:

Certain hormone-mimicking pollutants have major side-effects such as...

1- They alter brain function.

2- They alter our sex hormones keeping us sick, fat and depressed.

3- They alter our metabolic system and disrupt good gut bacteria.[70]

4- They can influence bone tissue.

5- They influence our circulatory system.

---

[70] Retha Newbold http://www.researchgate.net/publication/282130441_Endocrine_disruptors_and_obesity

Disruptors Harm Our Mind and Body

1- *The brain:* If there are toxins from pesticides and chemicals in the gut, they are also found in the brain. Foods with the highest pesticides content can be found in the green beans, peaches, corn, bananas, tomatoes, soy, pears, grapes, *milk* and beet sugar. *The Reaction*: The brain is disrupted by pesticides causing nervous system damage.[71]

2- *The lymphatic system:* An abundance of industrial and agricultural pesticides and chemicals have been linked to lymphoma risk. When a toxin enters the central nervous system the lymphatic elimination process is affected.[72] When the lymph doesn't work properly, this can lead to obesity.[73]

Our lymphatic system has front row seats to the blood's circulatory system and the immune system. As found in Chapter 6 ,"We're not separate parts?" Researchers now know our brain is directly connected to the lymphatic system through the immune system. This means we can now implement a better plan for the prevention of Alzheimer's Disease."Neurodegenerative diseases (Alzheimer's) are associated with immune system dysfunction." [74]

---

[71] http://www.ncbi.nlm.nih.gov/pubmed/18032333 see also http://www.scielo.br/scielo.php?pid=S0100-736X2011000700009&script=sci_arttext

[72] http://www.nature.com/nature/journal/v523/n7560/full/nature14432.html

[73] http://www.ncbi.nlm.nih.gov/pmc/articles/PMC3026597/

[74] http://neurosciencenews.com/lymphatic-system-brain-neurobiology-2080/

3- *Our elimination systems*: Mercury exposure can cause negative effects on the kidneys, cardiovascular, and central nervous systems, plus, many other body organs.[75]

Mercury alters brain and body fluid. Back in the 80's, as a Dental Hygienist, my sister use to play with mercury in the office like it was silly putty. No one knew the ramifications of handling mercury with their bare hands back then. It has been found to be an endocrine disruptor *with a reaction* that is toxic to women's ovaries, linking it to ovarian cancer. It disrupts endothelial cells. There is no safe level of exposure. Endothelial cells, are considered an endocrine organ. These regulate blood flow, are found in the heart chamber, immune system, lymphatic system and more.[76]

4- The *hypothalamus works in harmony with the pituitary gland to balance hormones.* The Hypothalamus is part of the endocrine system and contributes to the regulation of sleep and weight. Atrazine, a commonly used weed killer, disrupts these processes. Atrazine has been found to contaminate our water supply and golf courses. Atrazine can even lower our IQ levels. About sixty percent of the U.S. is exposed to this toxin. *The Reaction:* It contributes to insulin resistance, and obesity, especially in tandem with a poor diet.

5- *Estrogen levels*: Red meat has been shown to increase a higher estrogen burden on the body and negatively affect

---

[75] http://www.ncbi.nlm.nih.gov/pmc/articles/PMC3395437/
    environmental mercury http://www.ncbi.nlm.nih.gov/pmc/articles/PMC3988285/

[76]http://www.ncbi.nlm.nih.gov/pubmed/12379270

gut microbiome.[77] Why is this important? *"Estrogen dominance" effect gut bacteria and Cholesterol levels.* Gut bacteria influence how we process estrogen. Estrogen levels need balance to prevent obesity and diabetes.[78] When healthy gut bacteria are disrupted, we may experience increased menopausal symptoms over a longer period of time. As in past chapters of this book, good gut bacteria is key to a healthy mind and body.

Menopause Health

Having healthy gut microbiome is an important part of going through the natural process of menopause with ease. I have clients that ask: "When going through menopause is it a natural process to gain weight in the mid-section?" The answer is: No. Weight gain in menopause means there's an imbalance in the body where the communication system is interrupted, mainly in the adrenal glands.

The first culprit is **sugar**. Sugar disrupts our adrenal glands and increases energy loss. Sugar makes menopausal symptoms more severe, adds unwanted weight gain, causes Candida, increases anxiety and depression, depletes calcium levels and causes communication imbalances within the body.

The second culprit is **stress**. When we're under stress, our hormones are disrupted, causing weight gain, inflammation and high cortisol levels. Prolonged stress, and high cortisol levels leads us into high blood sugar levels. Stress has a direct relationship with insomnia.

---

[77] http://www.ncbi.nlm.nih.gov/pmc/articles/PMC3800670/

[78] http://www.ncbi.nlm.nih.gov/pubmed/12086946

A Bite Size Step:
For menopausal health, decrease alcohol consumption and
improve exercise and sleep habits.

Science Claims

Science Daily claims women nearing menopause have
higher levels of a brain protein linked to depression.
(MAO-A) They continue with: *"women may need earlier
intervention using HRT."*[79] HRT is a hormone replacement
therapy, and may increase your risk for breast cancer.

Do we really need HRT at a younger age?

First: What they failed to mention how a junk food
diet, sugar cravings, *acetaldehyde*, endocrine disruptors and
insomnia are related to higher brain protein in menopausal
women. (Acetaldehyde include synthetics, perfumes and
dyes)

Second: Some women use Botox for wrinkle control.
The botulinum toxin can move from the face into the brain
and damage brain cell proteins.[80]

Third: Mental function and brain proteins improve
with exercise and so does serotonin levels.

---

[79] http://www.sciencedaily.com/releases/2014/06/140604203159.htm

[80] http://www.jneurosci.org/content/28/14/3689.full

Fourth: The brain is made up of fat, Cholesterol, water, and cell proteins. When we have toxicity from free radicals in the body, these contribute to proteins and DNA injury.[81]

Logic tells us, if HRT contains bad science and increases cancer risk, then HRT doesn't improve health.[82]

Some Helpful Tips

We can stress-less by paying attention to what disrupts our adrenal glands. The spice turmeric demonstrates protective abilities in the communication systems of our mind and body. This spice can help alleviate depressive symptoms with menopause.[83] Turmeric can be added to soups, turkey rubs, smoothies, casseroles, fish dishes and more. Apple cider vinegar can help decrease cravings.

BPA's are considered a synthetic estrogen. These disruptors have been linked to serious health problems such as early puberty, brain and heart disorders, and prostate and breast cancers. The chemical companies convinced us BPA-free products are better. Unfortunately, these BPA-free products can still contain harmful chemicals.[84]

---

[81] http://www.ncbi.nlm.nih.gov/pmc/articles/PMC4350122/

[82] http://www.theguardian.com/commentisfree/2010/sep/18/bad-science-medical-ghostwriters

[83] http://www.ncbi.nlm.nih.gov/pmc/articles/PMC2929771/

[84] http://time.com/3742871/bpa-free-health/

*Disease occurs when your body
can't remove an abundance of toxins,
regardless of whether you're thin or fat.*

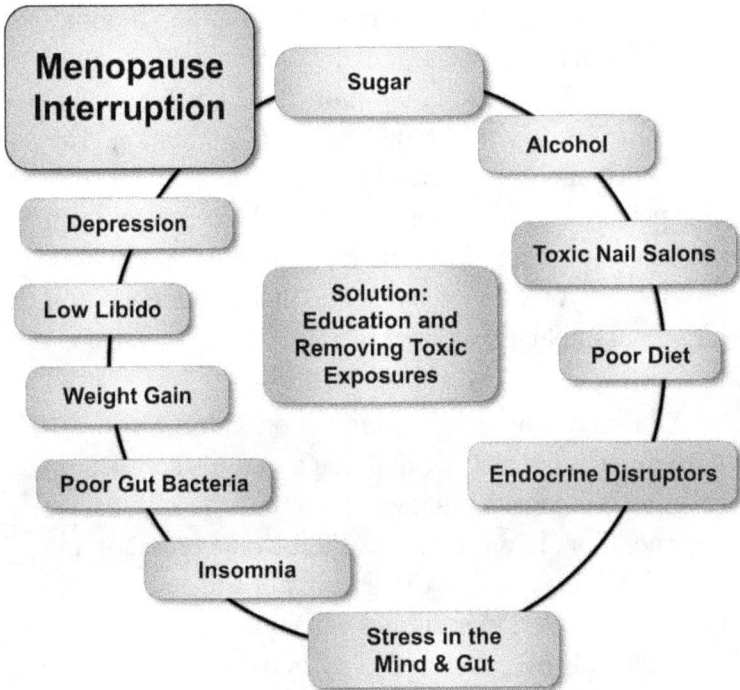

Menopause Interruption

Sugar

Alcohol

Toxic Nail Salons

Depression

Low Libido

Solution:
Education and
Removing Toxic
Exposures

Poor Diet

Weight Gain

Poor Gut Bacteria

Endocrine Disruptors

Insomnia

Stress in the
Mind & Gut

Endocrine Disrupters in Fibrotic Disorders

Fibrotic Dis-eases likely accounts for forty-five percent of American Deaths per year. Fibrotic disorders can be linked to toxins that can cause hormonal imbalances. In today's world, our internal and external environment is becoming more toxic. Additionally our nutritional levels are becoming more depleted increasing inflammation. The cause? An already tox-sick body tends to be more self-destructive. Fibrotic disorders can be linked to toxins that can cause hormonal imbalances.

But did you know women and men experience fibrotic hormonal imbalances under the guise of many other disorders?

Fibrotic Disorders are found in our brains in Alzheimer's disease, in our colon as Colitis and IBS, in our lungs as Pulmonary Fibrosis, in our eyes as Macular Degeneration, in our breast as Fibrocystic breast, in our heart as Cardiovascular disease, in our skeletal system as Osteitis Fibrosa and in tissues as Diabetes. "Inflammation and tissue fibrosis occur variably in tissue at different stages of diabetes complications."[85]

---

[85]http://www.ncbi.nlm.nih.gov/pmc/articles/PMC2515418/

74

Seven Fibrotic Disorders ~ You Can Prevent

1. *Breast:* Many toxins can be considered influential in the fibrocystic breast, such as synthetic hormones in our environment, along with rBGH hormones in our food supply and many endocrine disruptors which mimic estrogens that can encourage the proliferation of this condition.[86] They are called Xenoestrogens. They have been linked to pancreatic cancer as well. They are found in our water supply, food, soil, and many of the products you know and trust in your home.

2. *Osteitis Fibrosa:* Bone is a vitally important endocrine organ and endocrine disruptors can influence bone tissue. Xenoestrogens, an endocrine disruptor, can alter the systemic hormonal regulation of the bone remodeling process and the skeletal formation. This can cause inflammation. "The body's response to chronic inflammation can contribute to osteoporosis by way of elevated cortisol levels."[87]

3. *Colitis and IBS:* True health begins with a healthy gut environment. An imbalance will lead to fatigue, affect the body's ability to absorb essential minerals and nutrients, and hinder the repair of damaged cells while creating inflammation. A Leaky Gut may be implicated as a primary contributor to Crohn's, colitis and irritable

---

[86] http://www.ncbi.nlm.nih.gov/pmc/articles/PMC3759935/

[76]-http://www.ncbi.nlm.nih.gov/pubmed/21995947

bowel syndrome.[88] In fact leaky gut is directly linked to autoimmune disease. [89]

4. *Liver Fibrosis:* Sugar and alcohol are endocrine disruptors. These exacerbate liver fibrosis.

5. *Myocardial Infarction:* (fibrosis) is increased by high blood sugar levels.[90] We have a blocked communication system with junk foods, gluten, alcohol and sugar at the very core. These toxins can block the necessary systems in the body from working together.

6. *Macular Degeneration:* Disruptions found in the body from poor gut bacteria can be linked to disruption to the macula. Studies have shown that photochemical retinal injury is attributable to oxidative stress.[91] Oxidative Stress is a contributing factor in aging, hinders oxygen levels, and increases free radicals. What causes Oxidative stress? Bisphenol A, smoking, statins, a sugar habit, and countless other endocrine disrupting chemicals that are considered mitochondria poisons. [92]

---

[88]http://www.ncbi.nlm.nih.gov/pmc/articles/PMC4303825/

[89]www.ncbi.nlm.nih.gov/pubmed/22109896

[90]http://www.ncbi.nlm.nih.gov/pubmed/21348814

[91] http://www.ncbi.nlm.nih.gov/pmc/articles/PMC3392472/

[92]http://www.ncbi.nlm.nih.gov/pubmed/12634104

7. *Alzheimer's:* Studies show obesity, a high sugar diet and toxic vegetable oils can be destructive to the brain, and are linked to Alzheimer's disease. Inflammation in the gut and brain plays a role in Alzheimer's disease. When we don't pay attention to how we feed our body, it is quite common that we also don't pay attention to feeding our brain.

A Bite Size Step: Food, toxins, and stress have everything to do with disruption of hormones. You can take a simple proactive "bite size step" today and remove one toxin a week.

Johna's Story

The year was 1986 when Johna began not feeling well, experiencing night sweats and irregular menses. She was told by her doctor she had an irregular pap smear, which was possibly a yeast infection. She was sent home with medications that only made things worse. Exhaustion set in and her skin began breaking out all over her body.

After that first episode, she saw the doctor every six months for Urinary Track Infections.

Johna started questioning her doctors diagnosis. Maybe something else was wrong, she thought. After four years of doctors and prescriptions, she was not healed. Questioning the doctors lead the doctors to label her 'depressed' and in 1990 was put on yet another drug, an antidepressant. Certain doctors even refused to see her again.

"I have seen fibroids cause increased UTIs because the fibroids can obstruct the outlet of the bladder and cause some urinary retention. If the urine sits in the bladder, it becomes a reservoir for infection." - William Parker, M.D.

In 1991 to everyone's amazement, Johna discovered she was four months pregnant and went full term to deliver a baby girl. In 1992 she went back to the doctors with yet another UTI. In 1995, she suffered serve pain in her intestines and doctors suggested she should have her gallbladder removed. However, it was decided after a second opinion to be a false alarm. In 2002 she was told to see a gastroenterologist, gynecologist and an oncologist after a UTI emergency room visit. The oncologist was trying to figure out why she was anemic. He couldn't. At that point the gastroenterologist diagnosed her with Gerd (an acid reflux disorder), prescribed medication and told her: "I'll see you every month." After a year, she found no relief from this medication.

Sinus infections or UTI's controlled Johna's life. Each time she received a new antibiotic. She was always struggling for energy and asked her doctor if he could run a vitamin absorption test to see why the exhaustion continued. He explained there was no such test, although it was protocol with celiac disease. He prescribed 50,000 units of vitamin D weekly for the next 3 months just in case. Through the next 3 months, Johna experienced enlarged tender breasts, unbelievable pain through her entire body and started to have incontinence.

> *The warning signs were there but*
> *no one was paying attention.*

Then came the back pain. A tremendous amount of pain in her lower back that brought her to tears. It felt like she had suffered an injury of some sort. Her doctor put her into physical therapy, which she would continue for the following year.

When she saw her primary care doctor again in 2013, he referred her to his preferred gynecologist. After all the testing and retesting was done, there it was, a 20 cm x 20cm x 16 cm fibroid. Her doctor informed her this fibroid could definitely be pinching a nerve in her back causing her so much pain. Surgery was the only option recommended. Furthermore he added,"Due to the stitches that would have to be used in order to close the hole left behind from removing the fibroid, he recommended the removal of the uterus." The real issue was that the fibroid had taken control of the uterus.

Before surgery, more medications (GnRh agonists which may cause bone density loss, and lead to osteoporosis [93]) were given to try to shrink the fibroid. The results: One may be shocked to find that after the removal of the fibroid and uterus, Johna still has back pain, incontinence and her energy levels flex daily.

---

[93] http://www.fibroidsecondopinion.com/treatment-for-fibroids/

A Bite Size Step:
Do you suffer from any fibrotic disorders? What natural
treatment or holistic practitioner do you use to support you
in your journey?

Clear and Present Answers

Johna joined my program after her surgery. Her only regret
was 'why did she wait so long'. No one asked what Johna
was eating, what could throw her hormones out of balance
or what was eating her. Smoking was never discussed. If
she had known she was sick from an abundance of toxic
exposures, she may have been able to choose a different
path for her mind and body health. Healing can begin when
we know the cause. A not so pleasant journey that began
almost 30 years ago ended with complications from
medications and surgery.

Medications that are considered endocrine disruptive
are: antidepressants, Gerd proton pump inhibitors,
Antibiotics and contraceptives. *Foods that are linked to*
uterine fibroids are sugar, rBGH milk, wheat, alcohol and
caffeine. Johna was sensitive to wheat and she was finally
diagnosed with celiac disease. (celiac-when gluten damages
the small intestines.)

There were clear warning signs of uterine fibroids.
Fibroids need blood to survive.[94] Five different doctors
including an oncologist couldn't find the cause for anemia.
Not one doctor addressed adrenal fatigue. Her symptoms
included swollen and tender breast, incontinence, missed
periods, anemia, UTI's, exhaustion, and back pain. These

---

[94] http://www.fibroidsecondopinion.com/fibroid-symptoms/

were all signs that fibroids were present. A Leaky gut developed after years of using Antibiotics. Studies show Antibiotics disrupt gut microbiome.[95] Looking back, Gerd was diagnosed in 2002 instead of the correct diagnosis, Leaky Gut Syndrome.

Remember when Johna experienced a rash all over her body in 1986? The skins microbiome was already disrupted. In 1995 the gallbladder was reacting to the abundance of Antibiotics from nine years prior.

In my program with Johna together we covered Candida and digestive health. (healthy foods and recipes, bone health, depression and endocrine disrupting chemicals for hormonal balance).

In Chapter 15 we talk about mitochondria damage and oxidative stress. There are certain antibiotics that increase oxidative stress that can cause the mitochondria to malfunction.[96] Johna's osteoporosis risk increased with her taking antibiotics that included fluoride,[97] along with medications prescribed for Gerd.

---

[95] http://www.ncbi.nlm.nih.gov/pubmed/21637027

[96]http://www.multibriefs.com/briefs/exclusive/long_term_antibiotic_treatment.html#.VfXcYWC29U4

[97]http://aop.sagepub.com/content/35/12/1540.abstract

What Women Need to Know

All of this may have been resolved with some basic questions and changes of diet, testing for estrogen dominance, and simple 'bite size steps' to remove daily toxic exposures. A Transvaginal ultrasound may have shown the fibroid at the beginning stages.

As found in Chapter 8, we talk about how the medical industry is based on symptom control. Symptoms can fall on deaf ears, when doctors don't have the time to listen to your concerns. These same 'deaf ears' can prescribe antidepressants when they don't know what else to do.

Some Helpful Tips

Our dietary habits are extremely important when the body is experiencing inflammation and hormonal disruption.[98]Allergies, inflammation and hormonal imbalances can go hand in hand.[99] And being Tox-Sick doesn't just happen, it's caused. Having inflammatory foods in our diet can bring on allergies, even if we've had them in our.diet all our life. There comes a point when the body just says enough!

Noteworthy: For uterine fibroids, ask your doctor to check for estrogen dominance.[100] The liver may be having elimination issues as well, because of exposures to an abundance of toxins such as Xenoestrogens or pesticides.

When people make radical changes in their emotional and physical life, only then can the body heal itself.

---

[98] http://skinhealthfromwithin.com/2014/02/18/inflammation-and-hormones/

[99]https://bitesizepieceseducator.files.wordpress.com/2015/02/allergies-linked-to-arthritis.pdf

[100] http://www.drlam.com/articles/estrogen_dominance.asp

Endocrine Disruption From Medications

If I were just to mention a few medications that are known endocrine disruptors, I would choose the most popular along with their side-effects. The end effect leaves toxins in our rivers and on tap. [101]

1- **Antibiotics:** Antibiotics can have several side-effects: one, being an abundance of Candida and two, interference with calcium absorption.

2- **Birth control pills:** Oral contraceptives can change insulin levels increasing a woman risk for diabetes.[102]

3- **Corticosteroids:** Mimics the effects of hormones and suppresses the immune system. Can increase risk for weight gain, swelling of the legs, HBP and ulcers.

4- **Chemotherapy**: Suppresses the immune system, affects the brain, digestive system, the skeletal system and sexual function. Can cause cancer in other parts of the body.

5- **Warfarin:** A blood thinner which can cause skin tissue death.(necrosis)[103]

---

[101]http://opensiuc.lib.siu.edu/cgi/viewcontent.cgi?article=1152&context=jcwre see also http://sciex.com/Documents/brochures/ms-cms_039263.pdf

[102]http://jcp.bmj.com/content/s1-3/1/19.full.pdf

[103] http://www.fda.gov/downloads/Drugs/DrugSafety/ucm088578.pdf

6- **Statins:** are found to be carcinogenic. [104]
Statins can increase the risk for heart disease and lower
sexual function. Today more men are using Viagra because
more men are prescribed statins. Viagra can in turn increase
the risk for heart disease and melanoma. (see Viagra and
melanoma risk[105])

7- **Both High Blood Pressure medications** and the use of
beta-blockers are associated with reduced lung function in
the general adult population.[106]

8- **SSRI's:** Antidepressants are never meant to be taken for
longer than 3-6 months. The side-effects can cause weight
gain and decreased serotonin levels. Some SSRI's contain
fluoride. SSRI's are linked to lung disorders,[107]increase
risk for drug-induced liver injury, elevated liver enzymes
and gastrointestinal hemorrhaging.[108]

9- "**Triclosan:** (an antibiotic) "often used in hand soaps and
hand sanitizers, can be absorbed through the skin as well as
by ingestion/mucosal absorption from certain dental

---

[104]http://jco.ascopubs.org/content/early/2015/01/20/JCO.2014.58.9564.full

[105]http://www.aboutlawsuits.com/viagra-144/

[106] http://www.ncbi.nlm.nih.gov/pmc/articles/PMC3090996/

[107] http://www.ncbi.nlm.nih.gov/pubmed/12212966

[108] https://www.mh.alabama.gov/Downloads/COMD/HealthMonitoring/
antidepliver.pdf see also http://livertox.nih.gov/Fluoxetine.htm

hygiene products containing triclosan."[109] We are sanitizing our hands into illness, thinking that we are healthy, when that is furthest from the truth. Triclosan is toxic to our liver.[110] Triclosan can also be found in city water, air filters and dehumidifiers.

10- **Acetaminophen** can play a causative role in endocrine disruption and, therefore, disrupt gut bacteria and increase liver toxicity and cancer.[111]

11- **HRT**: Has been linked to cancer. HRT does not prevent heart disease in women.[112]

12- **Sleep aids**: Has gastrointestinal side-effects. Studies show a sleep medication, to cause heartburn, stomach cramps and high blood pressure.[113]

Some medications and drugs have effects and penalties that we may find more painful then the dis-ease itself.

---

[109] http://www.catawbariverkeeper.org/EDCs

[110] http://www.sciencedaily.com/releases/2014/11/141117154612.htm

[111] http://www.ncbi.nlm.nih.gov/pubmed/21555699

[112] http://www.ncbi.nlm.nih.gov/pubmed/12385489

[113] http://drugabuse.com/library/the-effects-of-ambien-use/ see also http://www.ehealthme.com/ds/ambien/high+blood+pressure

You Can Rebuild Your Gallbladder Naturally

Gallbladder disease is more common than we may think. According to the American Gastroenterological Association, gallstones affect more than 25 million Americans, with one million new cases diagnosed annually.

Gallbladder removal is the third most common operation in the U.S.

The gallbladder stores bile. This bile acid is excreted during meals for us to digest fats. If the gallbladder gets clogged up with fungus and bile starts to back up into the liver, this can be the start of gallbladder disorders. The bile's job is to bleed down into the pancreas, causing it to excrete insulin. Too much insulin in the blood leads to hypoglycemia, which in turn makes our body store glucose, fats, and proteins that we don't really need.

Having a Cholecystectomy (Gallbladder Removal) and other surgeries may give an increased risk of developing cancer of other organs such as the breast, kidney or ovary, particularly if one has undergone more than one operation". ([114]) I have personally known 3 people that developed cancer after having their gallbladder surgically removed.

Let's look at a few causes:

1-Gallbladder disease and gallstones are almost always the result of poor nutrition. For example: consuming an

---

[114] http://www.ncbi.nlm.nih.gov/pubmed/1454760

abundance of sugary products, soft drinks, diet sugars, caffeine, alcohol, rBGH dairy and cheese, pizza, GMO's, pesticides, processed foods, junk food burgers or fried chicken, trans-fats, gluten, granola bars, bottled juices, white flour, corn, and a ton of processed and hormone filled red meats, all may contribute to the formation of gallstones. But that's only half the story. These foods are endocrine disruptors and play a causative role in inflammation which tends to keep the body in an inflammatory state. Solution... ditch the diet foods, trans-fats and products containing gluten. These can only make matters worst. A diet rich in green vegetables is recommended.

2- An oxidized form of cholesterol might also be responsible for gallstones. This means overcooked foods. This is especially dangerous when we cook using microwave ovens because of all sorts of nonexistent organics compounds not found in nature. A Swiss study found cholesterol levels to be higher within a week of drinking and eating food heated in a microwave. Chemicals formed from microwave cooking such as d-proline, a neurotoxin that may be responsible for Alzheimer's and Parkinson's disease. Solution.. remove your microwave! It's not so hard to do, I did it.

3- Eating or drinking foods that destroy COLLOIDAL DISPERSION may be what causes our body to precipitate forming gallstones. I've found the younger generation along with the elderly are consuming more junk canned foods, soda pop, and frozen dinners. It is well known that aluminum destroys colloidal suspension and causing precipitation resulting in gallstones. Eating foods deficient in magnesium and excess in calcium make it even worse. Solution...Avoid Denatured Foods in canned foods.

4- Environmental toxins are what influence our health the most. At publication, BeyondPesticides.org database lists 105 studies linking pesticides to several types of cancers. These include cancer of the bladder, bone, cervix, colon, **gallbladder**, liver, lungs, ovarian, pancreas, thyroid, melanoma, multiple myeloma, and neuroblastoma (cancer of the nerve cells). ([115])

5- Endocrine disruptors are also found in PCBs (polychlorinated biphenyl), which are neurotoxic and play a causative role in gallbladder disorders. ([116])

6- Researchers say here is an increase in gallbladder disease from using birth control pills. Recent concerns have been raised using drospirenone (primarily marketed as Yaz or Yasmin.) ([117])

7- Long-term antibiotics can also cause gallbladder issues.

8- Allergies to certain foods and medications can cause gallbladder pain, such as pork, eggs, coffee, oranges, peanuts, and more. You can avoid the above offenders and read about the side-effects from medications you may be using.

9- You can avoid "Eating Under Stress," which negatively affects the gallbladder.

10- Your liver can become impaired by thick bile buildup because of liver congestion and the gallbladder in

---

[115] http://www.beyondpesticides.org/health/pid-database.pdf

[116] http://www.ncbi.nlm.nih.gov/pmc/articles/PMC2791455/

[117] http://www.drugwatch.com/yaz/

relationship to Leaky-Gut. Avoid drinking alcohol. Leaky-gut can start at any age.

11- Obesity, Diabetes, Chronic Inflammation, Hypothyroidism, Hashimoto's and Insulin Resistance, can be other causes that may disrupt the gallbladder. ([118])

Gallstones can be reversed, but it's something that takes a bit of time. After all, they have been formed in your body over a period of decades, so it's not something you can get rid of overnight from a nutritional standpoint. True Health is never a quick fix. At the same time, I know some people experience extreme pain when passing gallstones. So obviously, one is looking for immediate relief. Hence surgery. However, there is a strong possibility that nearly all gallbladder removal surgeries are unnecessary. ([119])

Conclusion:

According to the National Institutes of Health, pain from gallstones results in about 800,000 hospitalizations and more than 500,000 operations each year in the United States. Unfortunately, the NIH doesn't give people a lot of information about how to actually avoid gallbladder problems. It's also critical to recognize that the gallbladder has an important function in digestion. So, if we just remove the gallbladder, we may be compromising our digestive health for the rest of our life.

----

[118] http://www.ncbi.nlm.nih.gov/pmc/articles/PMC2111403/

[119] http://www.newswithviews.com/Howenstine/james19.htm

A Bite Size Plan:
Taking care of our digestion system and gut microbes helps to keep our gallbladder healthy.

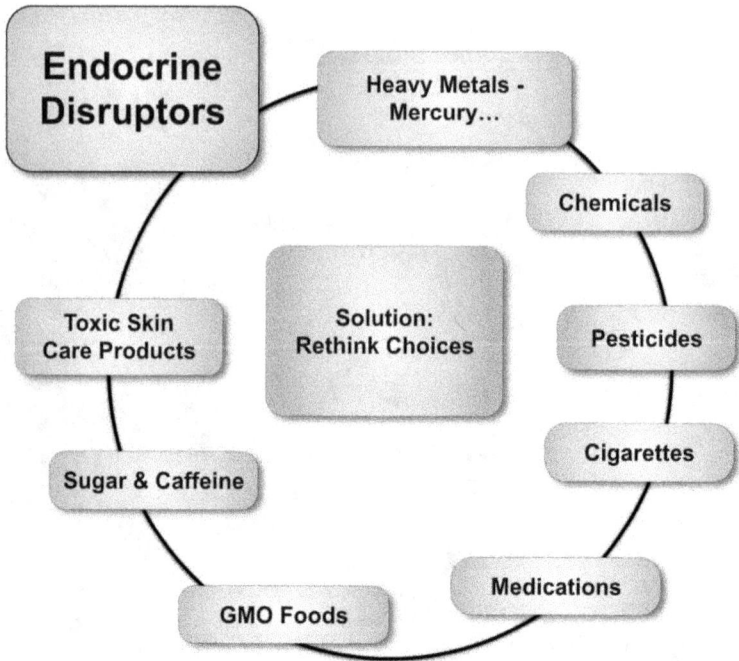

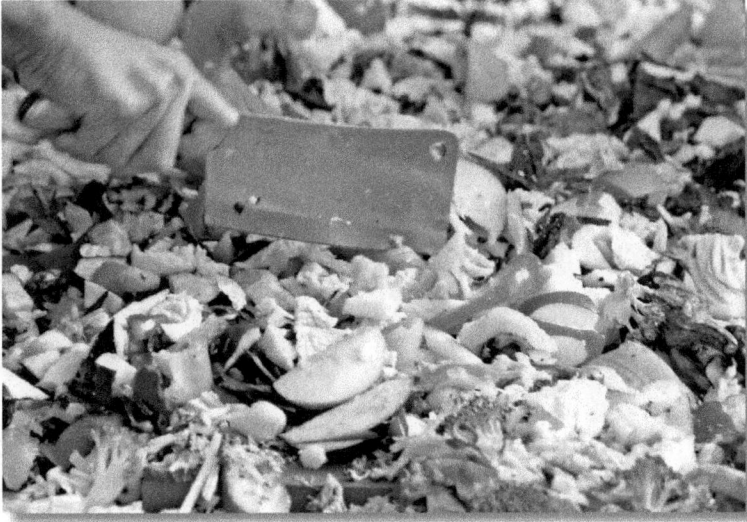

"The human body is no longer viewed as a holistic entity but rather as a grouping of separate parts and pieces."
Michael Culbert

Chapter 8

Food Works

Fast food. Rapid rise. Instant relief. Easy and immediate. Is this you?

In today's society we're always on the fast track - with little time for sleep or a sit-down meal.

However, if we don't take the time to care for our body, our body will force us to take time later, by becoming sick.

Sick is something no one has time for.

The modern way of treating illness is to find the afflicted body system or organ and send powerful drugs to it to manage it. Often the relief is quick, the results instant. The downside? Side-effects...

In Michael Culbert book: *Medical Armageddon*, "the physician's job was defined as managing symptoms. Eliminate the symptoms and you can eliminate the problem." Mr. Culbert is correct in his findings. Most insurance companies just want to know your symptoms when booking an appointment with the doctor.

If we believe we are just made of symptoms, then the whole world would be terminally ill. We are more than just symptoms. The body is integrative ~ always reacting and responding to everything that it experiences.

So what happens when we operate from a state of symptoms? James did just that.

The Artificial Industry of Symptoms

James is a gentle and kind man with a great sense of humor, in spite of growing up with three sisters. He was a tall and skinny kid in high school and lived on cheese, pasta, pizza, and desserts. As an adult, he didn't really change his eating habits. He started his day with coffee and ended it with more coffee. He almost never sat down for a real breakfast. In the afternoon, he snacked on processed foods and frequented fast food joints for lunch. Sundays there was always room for fresh cream cheese cannoli from a special NY Italian bakery after mass services. This particular habit began with his grandfather and was passed down to his generation.

James was busy holding down two jobs. At work there were plenty of available vending machines for him to snack from. Like most of us, he didn't understand the power of food, along with the power of movement. Arriving home in the evening he would pass out on the sofa not even making it to bed most nights. In hindsight, his body was storing more toxins than he could eliminate. He made an appointment with his doctor after a routine checkup and blood test at his job revealed his Cholesterol and Triglycerides were off the chart.

Stressed, lacking sleep and energy, he stumbled into his doctor's office, hoping for advice. His doctor checked his age, blood pressure and ran a blood test. He exclaimed: "Wow your Cholesterol is so high, you are a walking heart attack! James wasn't surprised. The doctor proceeded to write a script for statins. It took no longer than 15 minutes and James walked out the doctor's office thinking, finally, I'm going to feel better.

Following the doctor's orders, he took statins for two months. But he wasn't feeling any better, in fact, he felt worse. After just two weeks of taking statins, he became torpid and bloated, looking like he was pregnant with twins! He was not only worried about heart disease at this point because it ran in the family, but he was now concerned with diabetes. He wasn't fitting into his jeans anymore and didn't know what to expect next. That's when depression took hold.

Stepping in his wife said: "You need more help than those statins can give you. I'm going to call someone I know that can help us understand what's happening." Sara enrolled in my program to 'get the toxins out' and began reading my monthly newsletters. As it turned out she discovered the major 'side-effects' of statins were bloating, depression, and heart disease.

Immediately Sara had her husband read the information. He made the decision to stop the medication. Sara told him to start eating better and to stop eating out. (And he listened to her — THIS TIME.) She had bugged him about this at least eight times before in the last year. She insisted he take lunches with him to work. Additionally, she added more organic veggies to dinner time meals. They both began juicing in the mornings. Chips, gluten, coffee and sodas were a thing of the past.

Five months after removing statins and eating nutritious meals, James felt his body wasn't a stranger to him anymore. However, the bloating took much longer to dissipate.

Now, what?

The doctor wanted James to come into the office to see how the medication was working.

In the doctor's office another Cholesterol test was taken. The doctor said without lifting his head from the computer: "Great, the pills must be working. Your numbers are down!" "Actually no doc," James said, "I stopped the pills five months ago and I…" "What? You can't do that…the doctor screamed."

Almost two years have passed, and James is still drug-free. He started a new job where he is out and about getting more exercise and not stuck behind a desk as before. He has dropped 25 pounds. In addition, organic produce is more readily available in his neighborhood now. There are no more altered fats or toxic sugars in their home. Sara found through my program, that eating plants such as Brussel Sprouts which contain phytosterols and help balance Cholesterol.[120] She has even put together a "binder" with recipes for making healthy meals, included in my program.[121]

> *The body reacts the only way it knows how to, when toxins increase, elimination decreases.*

A frightening moment in time with a happy outcome. *The Reaction*: James suffered inflammation from eating junk foods and living on caffeine. When the body needs nutrients used for repairs, it must use what we give it, and

---

[120] http://www.ncbi.nlm.nih.gov/pubmed/15166807

[121] https://bitesizepieces.lpages.co/steps-to-get-toxins-out/

that is high-quality foods. High-quality nutrition ensures high-quality repairs.

Not everyone attempts to seek help outside of the norm. I am sure blessed that Sara found answers in my program. True health doesn't mean we'll never be without symptoms ever again. It means we'll be informed enough to know what our body is asking for at that particular moment. We might just need to slow down and take some time out for self-care or make new simple, sustainable changes. James and Sara both realized that symptoms are just a wake-up call. A call to make a healthy plan to take a positive action. Millions are spent to drive people in the opposite direction of what really works. Food Works!

As we evolve, avoiding toxic remedies can be made simple when we receive the support needed from a certified nutritional health coach.

I have discovered my program reaches more people because they're ready to take those necessary 'bite size steps' toward change that works.

"If it grows on a plant, eat it.
If it's made in a plant, skip it." Dr Joel Kahn

Some Helpful Tips

Inside the doctor's office, we may become concerned or frustrated when we watch the clock tic away for hours as we wait patiently to be seen by a doctor who rushes in and out without answering our questions. It leaves us wondering, "why do we receive better service at our favorite restaurant than at the doctor's office?" You may be shocked at the answer. The reason is, paperwork stands in the way of the doctor-patient relationship. This barrier is the result when government intervention supervenes our relationship with our medical provider.

A Recommended book on this subject is *The Digital Doctor* by Robert Wachter

Every organ and system in the body needs Cholesterol, especially our brain and endocrine organs. Every cell is made from it. Cholesterol is also the precursor of the five major classes of steroid hormones. [122] As you can see we can't live without Cholesterol, yet we believe it can make us sick. Why are there so many secrets surrounding the good, bad and the ugly of Cholesterol?

Are you confused? The truth is Cholesterol imbalances are created by poor dietary habits, sugar, and toxic exposures. These habits and exposures cause inflammation first. Inflammation is part of 'why Cholesterol becomes disrupted'.

I suggest reading "*The Great Cholesterol Con*" by Dr. Kendrick (contains 107 conflicts of interest, 70 directly with statin manufacturing companies)

---

[122] http://www.ncbi.nlm.nih.gov/books/NBK22339/

What Else Can Harm Cholesterol?

• *Heavy Metals.* "Mercury would classify as a heavy metal that negatively impacts Cholesterol levels."[123]

• *Medications* such as birth control pills or Antibiotics can wreak havoc in the gallbladder and can be linked to disrupting Cholesterol levels.[124]

• *Statins.* "Nearly 44 billion people have Alzheimer's disease."[125] Alzheimer's is inflammation in the brain. Could this be because of the frequent and widely prescribed use of statins?[126]

---

[123] http://www.westonaprice.org/health-topics/health-hazards-of-mercury/

[124] http://www.ncbi.nlm.nih.gov/pubmed/26129950

[125] http://www.alzheimers.net/resources/alzheimers-statistics/

[126] http://www.ncbi.nlm.nih.gov/pubmed/21981838 see also http://www.ncbi.nlm.nih.gov/pubmed/14574624

Myths or Truths About Cholesterol:

- The body is incapable of making hormones without Cholesterol. High Cholesterol means there is inflammation present. (T)

- Every organ and system in the body needs Cholesterol. Without Cholesterol our testosterone and cortisol levels are not adequate. (T)

- Our brain needs Cholesterol. (T)

- Our immune cells and our digestion rely on Cholesterol. (T)

- Both the liver and intestines are collaboratively involved in the regulation of whole- body Cholesterol balance. (T)

- We need statins to lower our Cholesterol levels. (M)

- Statins can cause an increased breast cancer risk. (T) [127]

A Bite Size Step: Find a plan that works for you to reduce sugar, heavy metals, and processed foods.

---

[127] http://blog.drbrownstein.com/statins-increase-breast-cancer-by-over-200/

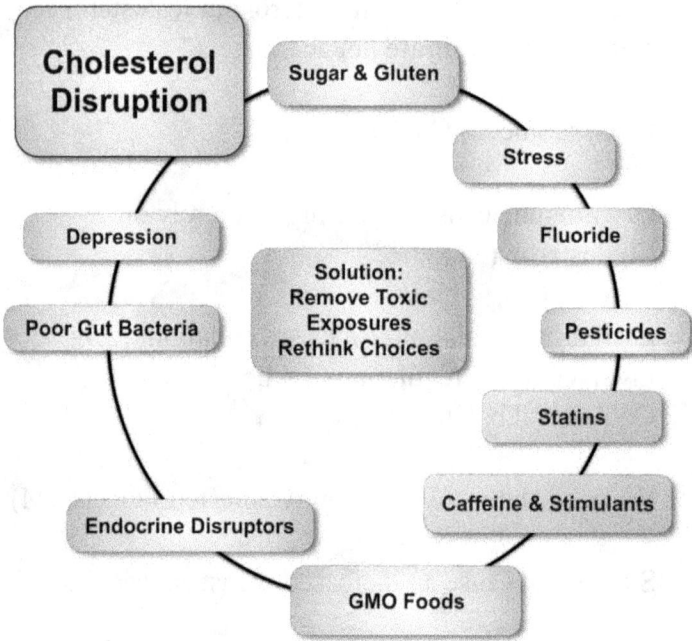

How to Order Healthy When Eating Out

When my clients complete their programs with me, they usually ask: "How do I find healthy options when ordering out?" Here are some helpful tips below.

Road trips can be challenging when looking for healthy restaurants, even for me. Since restaurants cater to the majority, the majority have developed decades of unhealthy eating habits. Most restaurant menus consist of processed foods, tons of buns, and animals raised through the massive industrial food production industry. The GPS software that conveniently guides us to our destination these days does not have the option to search for vegan, raw foods or organic based restaurants along our great highways. When we type in "healthy restaurants" or "salad bars," we find fast food and chain restaurants with few exceptions. Salad bars are healthy, right? Certainly one may think so; however, finding a healthy salad bar along the highway with produce that is sourced from organic growers is next to impossible. Most salad bars look plastic to me, almost surreal. Aside from the pesticides and chemicals used in food production these days, salad bars are sprayed with chemicals to keep them looking fresh while sitting in the open air. Salad dressings are usually not prepared fresh and can contain unwanted chemicals.

A healthy road trip requires <u>avoiding</u> the fast food traps, such as fried chicken and shrimp, burgers, fast food franchises, and oriental buffets loaded with MSG and heavy oils.

Personally my search includes healthy food preparation as well. My red flags are dirty floors, unwanted pesticides and hormones in and on foods and rapid cooking in microwave ovens. One restaurant I visited advertised healthy food, but when I arrived, they only used a microwave. Imagine, they didn't have a big enough kitchen to cook in!

My advice would be: Begin by knowing what foods you won't eat. Know yourself and know what it takes to remain healthy. Try a restaurant serving foods that are known for being fresh and vegan-friendly. They know how to make colorful fresh salads or cook vegetables (without turning them into mush) and they offer more options for organic ingredients.

I would also look at the quality of a restaurant and not the quantity. Believe it or not, good restaurants will work with your special dietary request. I visited one Italian restaurant in NY with my sister. She said I could inform the chef of my special needs. I ordered a plate of grilled Italian vegetables in a small amount of extra virgin olive oil, fresh spices, garlic, and herbs. I was pleasantly surprised to see this colorful plate presented to me, just the way I envisioned it.

When ordering water at a restaurant: Order filtered water instead of tap water. Tap water can contain an array of undesirable chemicals including fluoride, medications and chlorine. Nasty stuff! A healthy restaurant will automatically give you a carafe of filtered water at your table.

Positive Food Choices

Here are some examples of foods with color that can be prepared at restaurants specializing in international cuisine.

Indian

Colorful vegetable non-dairy or coconut curry, or eggplant and fresh garlic and spices.

Italian

Look for the restaurant that makes real foods, no frozen, and no hormones in meats and cheese. If you order chicken or meat, make sure you know how it was raised. Ask if it was grass-fed. Forget the pasta and enjoy grilled veggies with fresh garlic and herbs. Check the menu for other grilled options such as wild salmon.

Japanese

Vegetable sushi roll (no raw fish), seaweed salad, organic wakame and cucumber salad, organic miso soup.

Thai

Coconut vegetable and quinoa dish. Wild salmon and vegetable dishes. Nori veggie wraps.

Middle Eastern

Organic Millet or Organic Rice w/ raisins, garlic hummus, OR baba ghanoush OR fresh tabbouleh salad with fresh garlic.

Mexican

Guacamole (non-dairy), grilled veggies and salsa (no vegetable oil), wild fish tacos wrapped in lettuce leaves, baby green salad (no iceberg), black bean soup with fresh spices to take it up a notch. Avoid all creamy salad dressings.

Raw and Vegan

Mornings are easy with fresh made smoothies and fresh pressed vegetable juices.

Everything is gluten, soy, and dairy-free. You can make your own dehydrated seed crackers with almond butter, or beautiful salads and vegetable wraps. Include a homemade fresh salad dressing.

American

Collard wraps include a choice of the following inside ingredients: grilled portobello mushrooms and wild salmon, fresh tomatoes, zucchini, carrots, bean sprouts, cucumbers, and fresh herbs.

Dinner may include: Baby greens, kale or spinach salad with lemon, apples, and nuts, OR homemade veggie soup (lentils) with homemade vegetable stock (no MSG stock), OR a grilled veggie plate with Brussel Sprouts and bits of raw cashews, OR organic quinoa topped with green and red veggies. As always, skip the caffeine and sugary dessert!

So relax! Don't have reservations about reservations. We can all make healthy choices.

When we fix our relationship with food, it becomes second nature. It also becomes easier, delicious and less stressful. The results: we feel stronger, healthier, more confident and more peaceful with our decisions. Now see how well you sleep.

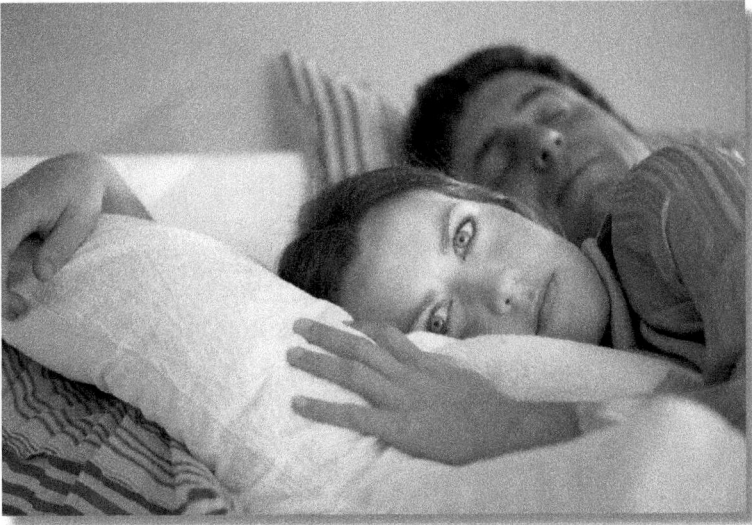

"If you can dream it, you can achieve it." Zig Ziglar

Chapter 9

Kicking Insomnia In The Gut

Having good sleeping habits is a very big part of health. Yet over sixty percent of the adult population suffers from insomnia. I think it's time to shed a little light on this dark subject and show just how insomnia can affect everything we do. Knowing there's always an action and reaction in the body when it's experiencing insomnia we can actually see the relationship between insomnia and obesity, depression, weight gain, endocrine disruption, Alzheimer's, disease, and insulin resistance.

Sleep is a restorative process and this means that when we sleep, we release toxins.

If we don't sleep well and keep running on empty, it's like crossing our fingers when driving through a red light. This is never recommended for optimal health!

If we're like most, we may feel like we never get enough sleep, or we could sleep nine plus hours a night. We may wake up tired with a groggy hangover feeling at 2am and can't go back to sleep. This can be our wake-up call that something's awry.

The body is always working when we sleep

- Every system in the body eliminates toxins. Even as we sleep, the brain eliminates toxins.
- The liver is usually detoxing at 2 am. In addition, the kidneys and liver rebuild at night when we sleep.
- When we sleep, imagine 'tiny elves' working round the clock assisting our elimination systems. If these are not functioning properly, sleep can be disrupted.
- Sleep is not a passive event, but rather an active 'volleyball tournament' involving characteristic physiological changes in the organs of the body.
- When the elimination systems are impaired, we have weight gain, insulin resistance, insomnia and disease. (And maybe a few dead elves)

Taking a sleeping pill is a quick fix, but never the answer. We can end up increasing our toxic load, risking disease, addiction, and premature aging.

Chances of Weight Gain
when we don't sleep

• When we don't sleep well, the body holds onto toxins and weight. The elimination systems are thrown out of balance and gut bacteria is disrupted. As a result one may experience constipation and/or skin issues.

• "More serotonin is found in the gut than the brain and it regulates a wide variety of brain functions and behaviors such as circadian rhythms to assisting the hormone, leptin."[128]

• Sleep balances leptin and ghrelin, the hormones that send signals to start and stop eating. Hunger cues are thrown off track when we don't get enough sleep.

• With chronic insomnia, the body experiences cravings. When using the computer late at night, we increase cravings, insomnia and deplete vitamin D levels. Increasing cravings can lead to weight gain 'and some gremlins destroying our kitchen.'

• Prolonged stress impacts the adrenal gland that, in turn, impacts sleep function. High cortisol levels in the

---

[128] http://www.nature.com/scibx/journal/v2/n37/full/scibx.2009.1396.html

evening are linked to insomnia.[129] High cortisol levels may add to eating disorders.

There are Immune System Consequences when we don't sleep

The brain has an immune system that is connected to the body's immune system. Stimulation and communication takes place between our immune system and our gut, with eighty percent of the immune system being found in the gut. There is a significant interaction between sleep and the immune system (or systems), and 'restorative' sleep is needed to maintain both gut and brain immunity.

The catch 22?

Without good immunity we can suffer sleep deprivation. "Chronic sleep deprivation maybe linked to causing an increased mortality rate."[130]

[129] http://www.researchgate.net/publication/ 11441316_Neuroendocrine_dysregulation_in_primary_insomnia

[130] http://www.ncbi.nlm.nih.gov/pmc/articles/PMC3132857/

What is linked to Insomnia?

Considerable research has linked endocrine dysfunction and sleep dysfunction as 'toxic family members.'[131]

Endocrine disrupting chemicals disrupt hormone levels and can keep us sick, fat and depressed in several ways. These include:

• Chemicals in our diet can play a causative role in depression. Depression is associated with insomnia. This is another issue powerfully connected to the way the body acts and reacts when exposed to toxins. Toxins that play a role in depression are connected to unwanted weight gain, making obesity risk higher if taking an antidepressant.

• Our sex hormones influence circadian function. When we have depleted testosterone, we can equally have a disrupted sleep cycle. What disrupts testosterone levels, is a high sugar diet.

• Sugar is 'the evil stepmother' tempting us as she plays her role in the endocrine disrupting process. Endocrine disrupting chemicals are linked to obesity, heart disease, metabolic syndrome, and diabetes.[132] Excessive consumption of sugar, poor gut bacteria and diabetes are offenders in insomnia.

[131] Institute of Medicine (IOM) Committee on Sleep Medicine and Research, Colten HR and Altevogt BM (ed.), Sleep Disorders and Sleep Deprivation: An Unmet Public Health Problem, Washington, DC: National Academy of Sciences, 2006.

[132] http://www.ncbi.nlm.nih.gov/pubmed/21054169

• Mercury alters brain and body fluid and is an endocrine disruptor. It's the 'silly putty' in fish, high fructose corn syrup, beaching creams, lipstick, and dental fillings. "Mercury in all forms poisons cellular function. In addition to brain disruption, metallic mercury is also deposited in the breast, adrenals, liver, kidneys, skin, sweat glands, pancreas, lungs, and prostate."[133] Mercury disrupts all elimination cycles.

• Statins are one of the many medications 'with a tooth fairy on the sideline' that can interrupt hormone levels and cause insomnia. Insomnia was reported with a higher use of statins.[134]

• "A morning cup of sadness" (as quoted by Jon Stewart) stays with us all day and into the night. Caffeine is an endocrine disruptor. Coffee adds to an acidic gut environment, disrupts the immune system, adrenal glands and sleep patterns.

• So what about that cake we bought yesterday? Wheat acts as an endocrine disruptor and is just as disruptive as sugar. It can have a negative effect on the nervous system, immune system, and digestive system. Therefore, wheat can affect the brain cells and lead to an acidic internal environment.

---

[133] http://www.hindawi.com/journals/jeph/2012/460508/

[134] http://www.ncbi.nlm.nih.gov/pubmed/19026028

We can experience Metabolic and Endocrine
consequences when we don't sleep

Insomnia plays 'the wicked witch' when it comes to the metabolic and endocrine systems. Along the same lines, experimental studies have pointed toward an association between sleep deprivation and the development of serious metabolic and endocrine consequences, particularly diabetes,[135] and heart disease. So we can safely say insomnia is linked to the development of glucose intolerance and hypertension.[126]

The Brain is the Most Important Organ
in Our Body

Every thought and action we have is controlled by our brain. Without a good night sleep, we increase the body's toxic load for the following day.

So my question would be "is opening the door to this 'trash pickup' at night valuable?" And the answer is a BIG YES! A good nights sleep releases toxins.

If we find our daily lifestyle includes an abundance of toxins that are secretly having an affair with our circadian rhythms, it may be time to make a "B line" for change.

"We find people in various stages of sleep. And then
we get to tap them on the shoulder and be with them
as they wake up to the full magnificence of life."
Sydney Banks

A Bite Size Step:
Good sleeping habits are essential. Ask yourself, are you
ready to sleep well?

Some Helpful Tips

A toxic and inflamed body can keep us awake. However I
found if we use stimulants during the day, the body can't
eliminate them fast enough in order for us to relax and
sleep in the evening. Enjoy your day stimulant-free and
junk-free.

Noteworthy: Make a plan to see a holistic dentist for
mercury removal in your teeth. Dr. Robert Gammal said
"Mercury from amalgam fillings has been shown to be
neurotoxic… and capable of causing immune dysfunction
and auto-immune diseases."[136]

---

[136] http://drsircus.com/medicine/cancer/mercury-and-cancer-research-dental-amalgams

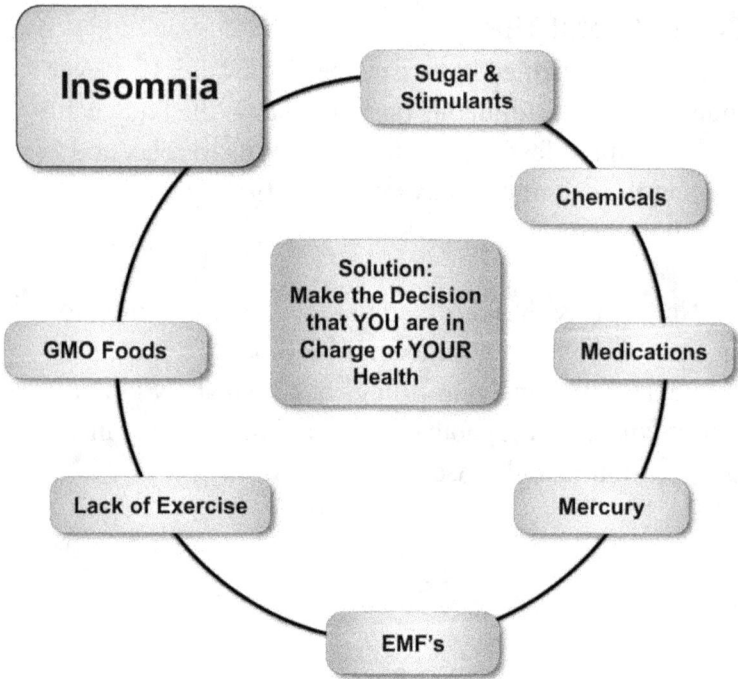

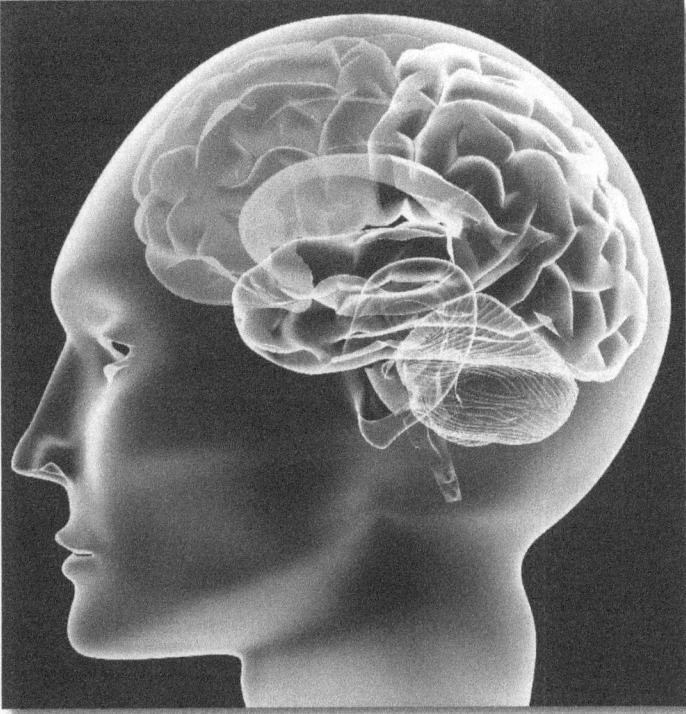

*Every muscle needs to be used regularly,
especially the brain!*

Chapter 10

Big Brain - Little Brain

Every thought and action we have is controlled by our brain. These include sleep, digestion, memories, movement and more.

"The brain directly communicates with the stomach and intestines (which is what we call the gastrointestinal system) through the vagus nerve." [137] Because of this we now know insulin resistance can begin in the brain first.[138]

Dr. Agnes Flöel said: "...even for people within the normal range of blood sugar, lowering their blood sugar levels could be a promising strategy for averting memory problems and cognitive decline as they age."

Research tells us that we can rebuild our brain with the foods we put in our gut. We can change its function and structure throughout our entire life.(Adapted from my life coach blog[139]) For instance, "if we are obese, we can have smaller brains," as said by Dr. Daniel Amen. When we are balanced and fit we have a balanced brain. When we invite health into our gut, we do the same to the brain. If we have a sedentary lifestyle, our brain will suffer.

---

[137] http://neurosciencenews.com/lymphatic-system-brain-neurobiology-2080/

[138] http://www.sciencedirect.com/science/article/pii/S0006295212003504

[139] http://www.lifecoachradionetworks.com/articles/2014/5/28/the?rq=we%20can%20change

There are habits we do way before age seventy that cause the brain to shrink! And these same habits trigger immune disorders.

- According to *Biological Psychiatry,* alcoholics tend to have smaller brains than nonalcoholics.[140] A study shows that brain size in alcoholics is also affected by their parents' drinking, even before the alcoholic's dependence begins.[141]

- Antipsychotics are documented as being linked to brain shrinkage as well as killing brain cells.[142]

- The brain needs Cholesterol. Depression, medications and a high-sugar diet causes inflammation and disrupts Cholesterol balance, paving the way to a smaller brain size.

- SSRI's are associated with and causing brain atrophy. (Selective Serotonin Repute Inhibitor)

- Insomnia decreases brain size [143] and undermines adrenal gland function.

---

[140]http://www.ncbi.nlm.nih.gov/pmc/articles/PMC1940091/

[141]http://europepmc.org/abstract/MED/17306776

[142]http://www.nature.com/npp/journal/v32/n6/abs/1301233a.html

[143]http://www.ncbi.nlm.nih.gov/pmc/articles/PMC1978381/

• High Blood Sugar levels are linked to a smaller brain size.

• Diabetes is related to changes in cognitive function and a smaller brain size. [144]

What Can Kill Brain Cells?

• Exposure to toxins can kill brain cells.

• Tobacco products, including cigarettes and chewing tobacco called NNK (pro-carcinogen), cause white blood cells in the body's central nervous system to attack healthy brain cells. [145]

• Ketamine, an anesthetic, has been linked to the death of neurons and neuronal toxicity. And, believe it or not, is currently being investigated as an alternative treatment for depression.[146]

• Taking steroids can lead to elevated levels of testosterone which in turn can kill brain cells.

---

[144] http://www.ncbi.nlm.nih.gov/pubmed/22933440

[145] http://www.sciencedaily.com/releases/2009/06/090623090400.htm

[146] http://www.ncbi.nlm.nih.gov/pubmed/19580862

- "Excitotoxins can excite cells to death." as said by Dr. Russell Blaylock. Aspartame can lead to neuronal destruction and damage by causing brain fluid to thicken.[147] Fluoride can induce DNA damage and cell death "cytotoxicity."[148] Fluoride can also be linked to Alzheimer's disease, and Dementia."[149]

- Oxidative stress is about free radicals that are highly reactive forms of oxygen have an ability to kill brain cells. "With increased oxidative stress, dopamine dies."[150] Anti-depressants also reduces dopamine levels. "Dopamine is a neurotransmitter in charge of the brains' reward and pleasure centers."[151]

- Chronic Sleep deprivation can cause cell death.[152]

- Chemotherapy kills brain cells.[153]

---

[147] http://universitynaturalmedicine.org/wp-content/uploads/Aspartame-and-Neuordegenerative_Diseases.pdf

[148] http://www.hindawi.com/journals/isrn/2012/403835/

[149] Fluoride: The hidden poison in the national organic standards by Ellen & Paul Connett Ph.D

[150] http://www.ncbi.nlm.nih.gov/pubmed/16475001

[151] https://www.psychologytoday.com/basics/dopamine

[152] http://www.thecrimson.com/flyby/article/2011/3/25/sleep-yoo-brain-study/

[153] http://www.urmc.rochester.edu/news/story/index.cfm?id=1312

"Every bite of food we eat broadcasts a set of coded instructions to our body that can create either health or disease." Dr. Mark Hyman.

Consuming a daily dose of toxins, chemicals, genetically modified foods and low fats alters our energy and frequency at the cellular level and can lead to early signs of brain disorders. Research tells us that a sick-brain is now quite common in age groups from 15-44.

A Bite Size Step:
Ask yourself: What are 3 things you can change in order to have a healthier brain right now? Go do it!

Some Helpful Tips

Our brain functions best when we include exercise as a daily habit. Eating curcumin helps with the damaging effects from fluoride.[154] Include these vegetables listed below that help release fluoride. (Garlic, onions, broccoli, asparagus, and tomatoes.)

---

[154] http://www.ncbi.nlm.nih.gov/pmc/articles/PMC3969660/

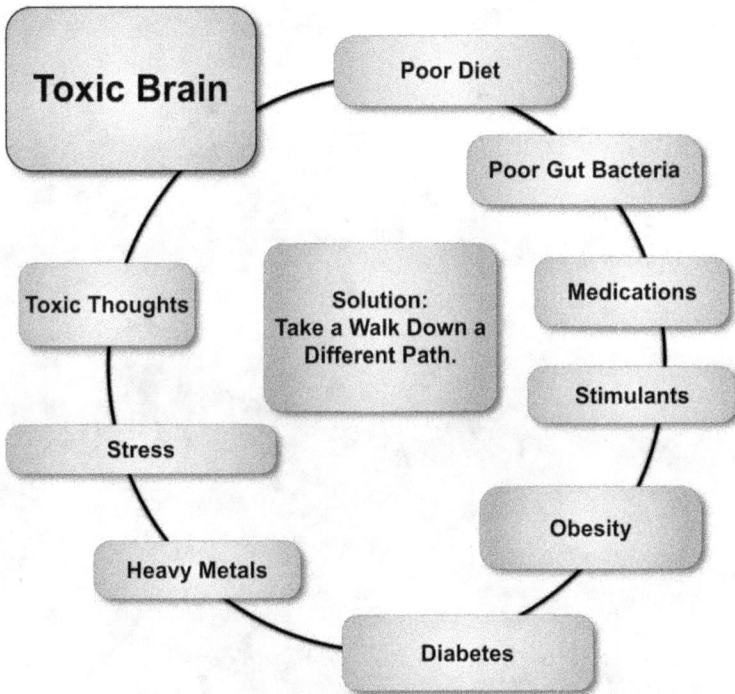

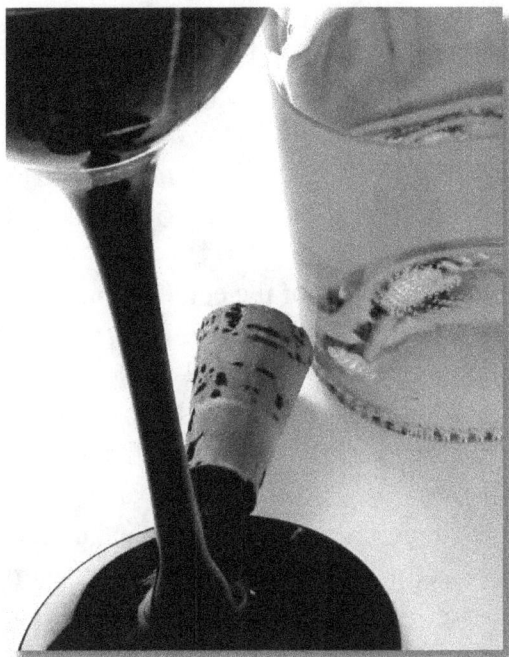

Our Skin is a Barometer of What Goes on Inside.™

Chapter 11

Hormones and Skin

Virtually every activity in our body is controlled by our endocrine system. Our skin is forever changing as it protects us and keeps us alive. However, without the correct information, we may fail to embrace the necessary changes that can keep us from appearing lifeless, old and toxic.

"The principle function of the epidermis is to regulate epidermal permeability and to act as a physical, chemical, and antimicrobial defense system."[155] Studies have shown that stress, hormonal disruption, and poor gut bacteria can impair the integrity and protective function of the epidermal barrier. (epidermis-the outer layer of skin)

Research suggest a poor diet causing skin infections can be linked to insulin resistance and liver disease, making cells less responsive which damages their ability to adapt. So we can safely say our hormonal system, when disrupted, can be the root cause of premature aging.

Eight Reasons for Premature Aging

Telomeres protect the end of our chromosomes. It is thought that shorter telomeres plays an important factor in aging. Below is a small list on what can shorten our telomeres.

- **An abundance of sugar and alcohol**: shortens telomeres and can lead to premature skin aging. A process called 'glycation' takes place with the introduction of sugars into the body, and this chemical reaction renders bodily tissues inflexible or damaged. Which cells are most vulnerable? Collagen and elastin

---

[155] www.ncbi.nlm.nih.gov/pmc/articles/PMC2045620/

is what keeps our skin firm and youthful. Once damaged, their depletion leads to wrinkles and sagging skin.

• **Poor choices of fats:** exert an inflammatory effect within the body that creates a stiffening of the arteries and constricted blood vessels. This can lead to less blood flow to the skin leaving skin older, stiffer, and more wrinkled. (my blog[156]) This is called Advanced Glycation End Products. There is mounting evidence that AGE's are caused by trans-fats, meats and processed foods, and implicated in diabetes and cardiovascular disease.

• **Unbalanced Cortisol levels:** When our cortisol levels are too high or too low, we increase oxidative stress.[157] "In women, psychological stress is associated with indicators of accelerated cellular and oxidative stress, telomere length, and telomerase activity."[158]

• **Insomnia**: When we lose sleep, our skin loses its chance to rejuvenate and rebuild.

• **Stress and over-eating**: shorten telomeres[159]

---

[156] http://skinhealthfromwithin.com/2015/05/27/foods-that-make-you-age-faster/

[157] https://en.wikipedia.org/wiki/Oxidative_stress

[158] http://www.pnas.org/content/101/49/17312.long

[159] http://www.hormones.gr/503/article/article.html

• **Triclosan**: is found in hand sanitizers. (Adapted from my blog on Natural News[160]) When used in hospitals, schools and grocery stores, triclosan is toxic to our liver.[161] Triclosan also contributes to issues of antibiotic resistance.

• **Formaldehyde**: is banned from cosmetics in both Sweden and Japan and is generally accepted as safe (GRAS) in the U.S. Formaldehyde solutions can be absorbed through skin, destroy skin's natural oils and is a carcinogen.[162] It is common to find formaldehyde in cosmetic formulations such as shampoo, sunscreen, mouthwash, perfume, conditioner, shower gel, antibacterial hand soap, nail polish and even products designed for children such as bubble bath and some baby shampoos.

• **Chemicals**: such as parabens, Sodium Lauryl Sulfate, Teflon, petroleum and propylene glycol in skin care products can play a causative role in aging, and weight gain. Some of these may actually alter the structure of the skin allowing additional chemicals to enter. The skin can absorb these 'Endocrine Disruptors' within 15 seconds. So we can safely say, habits that can lead to weight gain can also lead to premature aging. In fact, research has told us obesity will age us

---

[160] http://blogs.naturalnews.com/6-preventable-reasons-premature-aging/

[161] http://www.sciencedaily.com/releases/2014/11/141117154612.htm

[162] http://www.ncbi.nlm.nih.gov/pubmed/15140021

much faster than anything else.[163] Obesity is responsible for changes in skin barrier function and collagen structure.[164] Taking care of our skin requires us to reduce toxicities, chemicals, addictions, as well as obesity.

Some Helpful Tips

Skin Experts like myself say: "It's nutrition, and unhealthy habits and not our chronological age that determines how youthful we look and feel."

The skin's elimination process can become damaged by poor lifestyle habits. Reducing nutrient rich foods inside the body while adding in additional toxins on top of the skin, virtually eliminates nutrition to the epidermis. Choose organ foods and organic skin care.

---

[163]http://www.ncbi.nlm.nih.gov/pubmed/18982010/

[164] http://www.ncbi.nlm.nih.gov/pubmed/17504714

The Skin Reacts to Tattoo's

There are destructive and toxic ways we treat our brain, skin and other organs every day, without giving it much thought. I'm speaking of organ toxicity and tattoo ink. It seems millions of people old and young have received tattoos in their lifetime. But just like cigarettes years ago, the ramifications were never revealed until more and more people developed serious debilitating side-effects. In 1984 when my girlfriend received her first tattoo, I thought it was just a phase that she had to go through. Then she got another! As of a 2013 report, 45 million Americans have at least one tattoo.[165]

You might ask what is the reasoning behind the craving to get a tattoo? The answers range from it makes me feel sexier, rebellious or more intelligent.[166]

Today, studies are now warning us TATTOO INK is toxic.[167] How many signs have you seen posted on the toxicity and cancerous effects of tattoo's while you are receiving one? I have not seen one sign. In fact, there are no guarantees that tattoo inks or pens are sterile; however. New York tattoo studios will have single use needles in place by December 2015. And just when you think you've seen it all, someone decides to use blue tattoo

---

[165] http://www.statisticbrain.com/tattoo-statistics/

[166] http://www.statisticbrain.com/tattoo-statistics/

[167] http://www.thelancet.com/journals/lanonc/article/PIIS1470-2045%2806%2970651-9/fulltext

ink in their eyes! [168] I am amazed that one would deliberately want to harm their vision.

As you can see, the effects from tattoo ink in our skin can harm our immune system. Leaving me to wonder how such a painful and toxic experience can be so very addictive?

Five Ways the Body Cries After a Tattoo

1- After tattooing and wound healing, tattoo ink ingredients will stay in the skin or will distribute in the human body, particularly the regional lymph nodes.[169]

2- Scientist believe tattoo ink is a known carcinogen.[170] This means that cancer can be injected into your skin. Studies confirm that nanoparticles of titanium dioxide and carbon black ink are toxic.

3- Reactions to Tattoos can pose a health risk to the skin when exposed to UVA rays.[171] The introduction of foreign substances into the skin can result in a toxic or immunologic response. In addition to the transmission of

---

[168] http://www.dailymail.co.uk/video/news/video-1155367/Wow-You-need-BIZARRE-tattoos-display-Brazil.html

[169] http://www.ncbi.nlm.nih.gov/pmc/articles/PMC3966813

[170] http://www.dailymail.co.uk/news/article-2428867/Could-tattoo-cancer-Scientists-fear-toxins-ink-enter-blood-accumulate-major-organs.html

[171] http://www.ncbi.nlm.nih.gov/pubmed/20545755

infectious disease, reactions to tattoo pigments have also been a concern. These reactions include acute inflammatory reaction, and allergic hypersensitivity. Localization of skin disease in tattoos has also been documented.[172]

4- The liver can become inflamed when receiving a tattoo, linking tattoos to Hepatitis B and C.[173]

5- Finally, among those coincidental lesions reported from tattoo's are B cell lymphoma, melanoma, basal cell carcinoma, squamous cell carcinoma and non-Hodgkin's lymphoma.[174]

---

[172] http://emedicine.medscape.com/article/1124433-overview

[173] http://www.ncbi.nlm.nih.gov/pubmed/23315899

[174] dermatlas.med.jhmi.edu/derm/result.cfm?
OutputSet=4&BO=AND&Diagnosis=64

Some Helpful Tips

Tattoos are never good for the health of your skin. Now that you know there are several health consequences that can potentially harm your organs when receiving a tattoo, would you still want one?

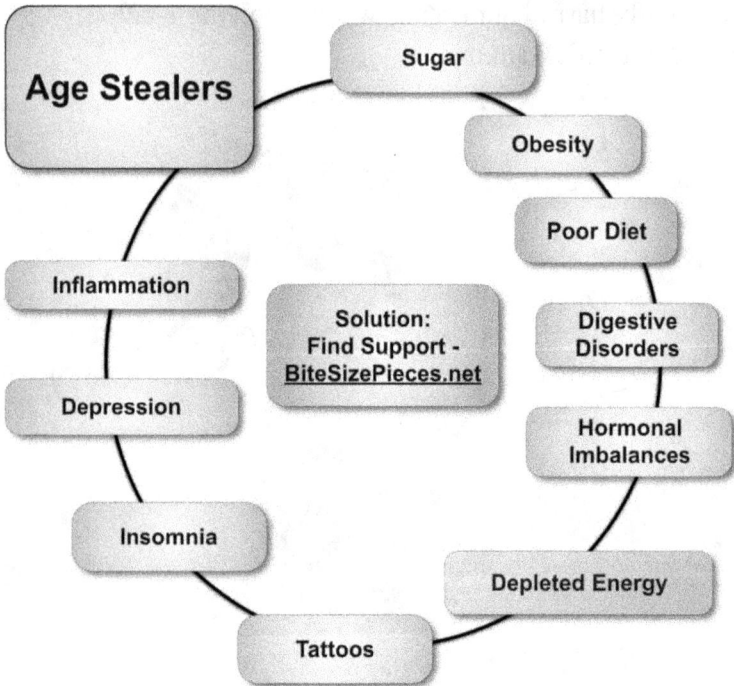

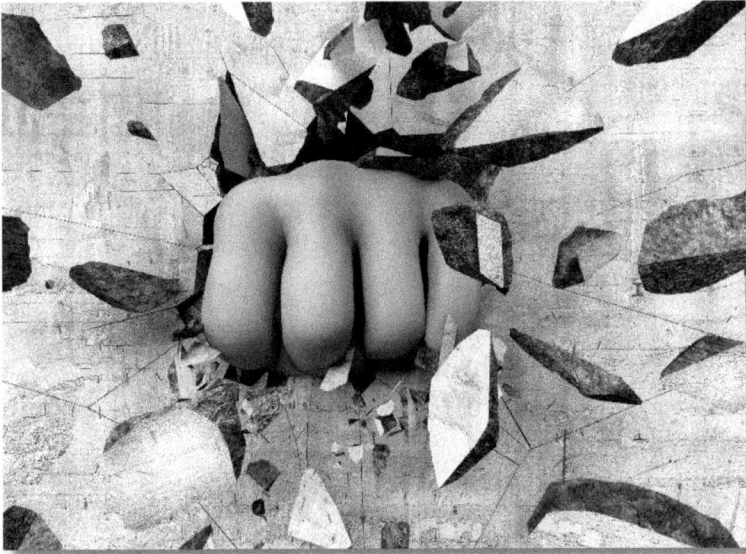

"Your wellness is determined by far more than your genes." Dr. Dean Ornish[175]

Chapter 12

Barriers That Prevent Health

---

[175]http://www.sott.net/article/220892-Why-Your-Genes-Dont-Determine-Your-Health

As you can see from the previous chapters, there are numerous barriers that prevent health.

The American Medical Association estimates that $575 billion is spent annually on the treatment of diseases or disabilities resulting from unhealthy, potentially changeable behaviors.[176] Imagine… we can feel so much better if we could just change one behavior. But what is that behavior and there's so much misinformation out there, where do we start? We can begin by taking the wool off our eyes.

First Barrier: Digesting Synthetics

A CDC report from July 2005 found that the bodies of Americans of all ages contain an average of 148 synthetic chemicals.[177] "Synthetic chemicals are not recognized by the body as food." [178]Thus, they are not absorbed properly in the body. Yet we eat them.

Uninformed and compliant we are a nation blindly ingesting synthetics. For over sixty years we have been exposed to the toxic effects of synthetics in our foods and vitamins. For instance: a fortified food is when a product is stripped of its nutrients, and synthetic ones are put back in. You can find these in processed cereals, breads, milk, orange juice, yogurt, granola bars and more.

––––––––––––––––

[176]http://www.medicalnewstoday.com/releases/197733.php

[177] http://stacks.cdc.gov/view/cdc/21808

[178] http://www.sunwarrior.com/news/natural-vs-synthetic-vitamins/

In the U. S., millions are found to be taking synthetic vitamin D. Synthetic vitamins can play a causative role in obesity.[179] So why is everyone's talking about how they need more of this sunshine vitamin?

Maybe we just don't understand what is depleting this natural vitamin that gets stored in our skin and liver. Obesity can block vitamin D levels along with chronic exposures to computer screen light, caffeine, sodas, sugar, statins, and ill health. Since the invention of toxic sunscreens, we have been able to effectively block vitamin D production in our skin. All these inhibit vitamin D receptors.

Because habits have caused depletion of this necessary vitamin we began adding in synthetics. However, high levels of vitamin D from vitamins may have side-effects such as heart issues![180] In addition, vitamin D in pill form may have "carriers" derived from GM corn sources. Misinformation fills the internet with how much of this synthetic vitamin is necessary. My thoughts are we can safely say "vitamin D2 and D3 is not the vitamin you may need from sunshine."

Some Helpful Tips

If you're vitamin D levels are low, loading up up on a cereal containing synthetic vitamin D, sugar and corn may not be the answer. Look at what can be depleting your vitamin D levels in the first place. A synthetic may throw off Cholesterol levels. Synthetic sources of Vitamin D are

[179] http://www.ncbi.nlm.nih.gov/pmc/articles/PMC3932423/

[180] http://www.ncbi.nlm.nih.gov/pubmed/25710567

irradiated ergosterol (yeast) and cholecalciferol. If the source is not given, it is usually synthetic.[181] I find the best source of vitamin D is sunlight. Shiitake mushrooms are also a good food source of vitamin D.

Other Vitamins in Question

1- The Adrenal glands negatively react from taking an abundance of omega 6 vitamins from GMO corn products or omega 6 fats from toxic vegetable oils. Omega 6 can lead us to increased inflammation. This in turn can depress our immune system.

2- Ascorbic acid may be a synthetic form of vitamin C, made from genetically modified corn. Your vitamin bottle may not use the word 'synthetic' on the label, even if it is. Synthetic vitamins do not act like whole foods when entering the body. A whole food vitamin C is made from Camu camu.

3- Women who take poor choices of calcium supplements for bone health may have an increased risk for heart attacks. Most people believe calcium supplements are relatively safe. We now know that high dosages of calcium supplements may adversely influence vascular health in both men and women.[182]

---

[181]https://www.organicconsumers.org/news/nutri-con-truth-about-vitamins-supplements

[182]Taken From -Researchers at the University of Auckland in New Zealand

4-"In 1989 thirty-seven people had died, and 1500 had become crippled eating L-tryptophan manufactured with genetically engineered bacteria by a well-known company. The evidence was destroyed."[183]

5-There are companies that advertise how we need more Glutathione in order to be healthy. However, Glutathione, in pill form, is not easily absorbed at the cellular level. "Glutathione is a very simple molecule that is produced naturally all the time in our body. The best glutathione comes from foods."[184] What depletes our glutathione levels is a question we need to be concerned with. A few habits include stress, inflammation, pesticides, sugar, chlorine, heavy metals, fluoride, tobacco, caffeine, MSG, and aspartame, just to name a few. Genetically Modified Soy also disrupts our glutathione levels.[185]

When we boost our vitamin C levels from organic food sources, we will boost Glutathione levels as well. Glutathione helps in the prevention of cancer, premature aging and heart dis-ease. Foods rich in Glutathione are cabbage, kale, asparagus and watercress.

---

[183]http://responsibletechnology.org/gmo-dangers/health-risks/L-tryptophan/cripplings

[184]Dr Mark Hyman "The UltraMind Solution"Book

[185]http://www.integrativesystems.org/systems-biology-of-gmos/

Disclaimer: There are times we need supplements, however, this information provided is a path to discover organic foods as a first choice, without synthetics, dyes, and toxic fillers.

Some Helpful Tips

"By eliminating inflammatory foods, and (inflammatory synthetic vitamins) and adding in essential nutrients from fresh, unprocessed food, we can reverse years of damage in the arteries and throughout the body." [186]

Feeding the body superfoods in turn, feeds our blood and circulatory system. Superfoods include Kale, Seaweed, Kelp, Broccoli, Green Algae, Hemp Seeds, Blueberries and more.

---

[186] http://www.sott.net/article/242516-Heart-surgeon-speaks-out-on-what-really-causes-heart-disease

Second Barrier: Pesticides and GMO's

In the 1960's Monsanto partnered with Dow Chemical manufacturing Agent Orange. In the years that followed, three million people were contaminated, and about one-half million died.[187] It is horrifying to think Agent Orange was brought back in 2014.[188] How crazy has our world become? History is doomed to repeat itself when lessons are ignored.

In 1992 the FDA granted genetically modified foods 'GRAS' (Generally Regarded As Safe) status.

Today the FDA claims health risk from GMO's are minimal to none, with these known toxins. This I have found not to be true.[189] Scientist say GMO's have unpredictable side-effects. This means it may take years before we find out what effect it has on our health.

"The year was 1996, where President Clinton gave the green light to Monsanto. GE-corn was planted in the U.S. Since then, there has been an increased rate of diabetes of 90%." [190] It wasn't long before Biotech companies owned 80% of our corn crop and about 95% of our soy crop. GMO corn and soy are found in everyday items such as processed, boxed and frozen foods, protein powders,

---

[187]http://www.wakingtimes.com/2014/06/20/complete-history-monsanto-worlds-evil-corporation/

[188]http://www.huffingtonpost.com/andrew-kimbrell/dow-chemical-and-monsanto_b_6041802.html

189 http://www.bibliotecapleyades.net/ciencia/ciencia_monsanto152.htm#Altered%20Genes,%20Twisted%20Truth%20-%20How%20GMOs%20Took%20Over%20the%20Food%20Supply

190 http://www.cdc.gov/mmwr/preview/mmwrhtml/mm5743a2.htm

sugars, corn chips, children's cereal, breads, ice-cream to meats, juices, alcohol, vitamins and more. Many years ago corporations have told us Agent Orange was safe and now they are trying to convince us GMO's are safe.[191] A government that is big on breaking up monopolies has a virtual monopoly between GMO's and itself, which includes Congress and White House involvement.[192] We live in a world where Corporate Profits rule while destroying our food supply seems meaningless.

It should be noted that Europe banned all genetically modified vegetables and fruits; however, the U.S. has not joined them. [193]

Are you being sold the disease as the cure?

Take a look at Acetochlor®. According to Samantha King, in her book *Pink Ribbons, Inc.*, "In 2000, AstraZeneca a pharmaceutical corporation, and the manufacturer of tamoxifen a breast cancer drug, was the leading producer of a GMO carcinogenic corn herbicide called Acetochlor®, that has been linked to breast cancer.[194] As of October 2015 according to AstraZeneca.com, AstraZeneca and Eli Lilly are working together on oncology research.

---

[191] http://www.responsibletechnology.org/10-Reasons-to-Avoid-GMOs

[192] http://www.globalresearch.ca/monsanto-controls-both-the-white-house-and-the-us-congress/5336422

[193] http://www.zerohedge.com/news/2015-07-24/it-cost-koch-brothers-only-299000-block-labeling-genetically-modified-foods

[194] http://pmep.cce.cornell.edu/profiles/extoxnet/24d-captan/acetochlor-ext.html see also https://en.wikipedia.org/wiki/Acetochlor

There's another piece to this toxic pesticide puzzle. 'Roundup Ready®' is known as Glyphosate®. This toxic poisonous chemical is not only on our food, we willingly spray it on our lawns. Most unsuspecting gardeners and non-commercial farmers are ignorant of the poisons they expose their body to on a daily basis. Glyphosate® wreaks havoc in the immune system and causes endocrine (hormonal) disruption.[195]

Glyphosate® is connected to chronic kidney disease.[196] Additionally there is a study showing Roundup Ready® causes cancer.[197] Where there's endocrine disrupting chemicals there's increased illnesses, depression, and weight gain.[198]

When Endocrine Disrupting pesticides play a causative role in depression,[199] then we can safely say GMO food products causes depression.

Glyphosate® is a organophosphate compound and is geno-toxic, as said by Professor Christopher Portier.[200]

---

[195]http://www.ncbi.nlm.nih.gov/pubmed/17486286

[196]http://www.gmoevidence.com/dr-jayasumana-new-research-supports-glyphosate-connection-to-chronic-kidney-disease/

[197]http://www.commondreams.org/news/2015/03/23/glyphosate-favored-chemical-monsanto-dow-declared-probable-source-cancer-humans

[198] http://www.ncbi.nlm.nih.gov/pubmed/24553011

[199]http://www.ncbi.nlm.nih.gov/pmc/articles/PMC1626656/

[200]http://sustainablepulse.com/2015/07/15/who-cancer-expert-glyphosate-is-definitely-genotoxic/#.Vb2IdGC29U4

That means it can damage our DNA. "Organophosphorus and carbamates residues (pesticides) are linked to depression."[201]

Glyphosate® negatively changes our gut bacteria which in turn makes us more susceptible to illnesses, brain disorders, [202]and is linked to non-Hodgkin's Lymphoma. [203]

Some Helpful Tips

For outside weed control, you can choose to make your own. Blend together a mixture of white vinegar, water and dish soap. Purchase a 2 gallon lawn sprayer and now you have an affordable, non-toxic weed control plan for your yard.

---

[201]http://www.ncbi.nlm.nih.gov/pubmed/17508698 see also http://poisonedpeople.com/organophosphate.pdf

[202]http://link.springer.com/article/10.1007/s00284-014-0732-3

[203] http://www.academia.edu/5838004/
HUMAN_HEALTH_ENVIRONMENTAL_and_ANIMAL_IMPACTS_OF_PESTICIDE
S_IN_GENERAL_and_ORGANOPHOSPHATES_IN_PARTICULAR

Third Barrier: Promoting Stale as Fresh

Think we're drinking fresh and natural OJ? Think again......

When shopping for fresh orange juice, I have found the phrase "squeezed from fresh oranges," is not the whole truth! Yes, I thought I was buying fresh orange juice for my family but, here's what I've found. The leading orange juice companies such as Tropicana (PepsiCo)[204], Minute Maid (Coca-Cola), and Florida's Natural (Citrus World Inc.)[205], tell us several stories. It's natural. It's pure and simple, and it's squeezed from fresh oranges. But they leave out the details about what they think freshly squeezed really is. The unfortunate reality is that it's anything but fresh!

In the 1980's Tropicana coined the phrase "not from concentrate" to distinguish pasteurized orange juice from the reconstituted concentrate brand. The idea was to convince us that pasteurized is a fresher, overall better product and so it cost more.[206] Put enough advertising behind a product campaign and anyone can convince the masses to believe a new version of almost anything.

However, little were we aware that it involved stripping the juice of oxygen, so it doesn't oxidize in large tanks in which it can be kept for a year. When the juice is stripped

---

[204]http://www.seegerweiss.com/law-practices/class-actions/consumer-actions/tropicana-juice-class-action/

[205]https://en.wikipedia.org/wiki/Florida%27s_Natural_Growers Wikipedia®

[206] http://www.macleans.ca/culture/fresh-from-the-press/

of oxygen, it's also stripped of flavor. Flavor packs are then added in and nutritional value is lost.[207] "Refrigeration combined with pasteurization and hermetic packaging can further increase storage life with minimum quality changes, but then the juice cannot be labeled fresh".[208]

Why pasteurize?....if drinking fresh is best!

The commercial juice industry is said to be a billion dollar industry. Corporations need more than a week of shelf life on their products. The protective agencies think that "fresh" poses risks and they need to kill off food borne diseases. They think GMO's will protect processed foods.[209]

However, pasteurization of orange juice kills any benefits of the food, and reduces nutrient content, leaving it a dead food less food. Pasteurization and thermal heat destroys important key enzymes. Enzymes carry out activities of metabolism. Kill the enzymes and we now have created a product harder for our digestive system to digest.

---

[207] http://www.macleans.ca/culture/fresh-from-the-press/

[208] http://www.fao.org/docrep/005/y2515e/y2515e09.htm

[209] http://www.fao.org/docrep/005/y2515e/y2515e09.htm

Are There Any Problems Drinking Processed Chemicals?

Just a few...

1-Processed orange juice may cause our bodily systems inflammation and increased allergies. A number of children are consuming orange juice every day in place of water.

2-Sugary beverages and sweets increase our risk for pancreatic cancer.[210]

3-Giving fake, lifeless orange juice to diabetics is ludicrous because sugar doesn't cure sugar- related disabilities. This practice can cause more harm than good.

Today there are several new alterations of our food system in the U.S. Genetically modified oranges are on their way to Florida and Texas. Really? Oh yes, these artificial oranges are supposed to be good for the farmers and the corporations, but little concern is given to our health. These will be oranges that are resistant to "citrus greening."[211] The EPA's gave its approval to Southern Gardens (related companies are Citrus World Inc, Dole Juice, Naked Juice, Tropicana, Tree Top and more) and plans to plant 150 acres in Florida and 50 acres in Texas.[212]

If we add a little humor to this 'Orange Juice Dilemma', one can say: "I just wanted a glass of fresh

---

[210] http://www.ncbi.nlm.nih.gov/pubmed/23368926

[211] https://en.wikipedia.org/wiki/Citrus_greening_disease Wikipedia®

[212] http://www.huffingtonpost.com/2015/05/14/gmo-oranges-citrus-greening-southern-gardens_n_7244858.html see also https://www.google.com/finance?cid=12863136

squeezed orange juice, but my government has strict regulations in place, and I have to buy dead food instead. The side-effects I can experience can lead me down the road toward diabetes, cancer, heart disease, walking hunched over with a cane, lost energy and Alzheimer's Disease." Not so funny after all!

Everyday people can be confused with thousands of ad campaigns promoting misinformation in what's truly healthy and what's not. If you've been deceived with fresh squeezed, you're not alone.

Some Helpful Tips:

Barriers can begin in our mind. Get in touch with your thoughts, opinions and lifestyle choices that are standing in your way of whole body health. Start the day with fresh whole foods. Calcium from fresh fruits and vegetables provide the body with electrical energy. Lacking energy can leave it's mark on generations to come.

However, all is not lost. You can tap into wellness. With the support from a coach, you can learn to ditch dead foods, work through stress and add in exercise in order to change your DNA. (see, The science of Epigenetics, DNA isn't your Destiny.[213])

---

[213] http://www.theverge.com/2013/12/13/5207640/the-shadow-genome-why-dna-isnt-destiny-epigenetics

Fourth Barrier: Deceived by Big Pharma

Scientific facts are found to be influenced by Big Pharma. This may prove dangerous to our health and are in direct violation of scientific standards. For example 40 thousand Americans died while using Vioxx, a pain relief medication with side-effects that caused risk of heart attacks and death. Scientific facts were not disclosed, and while people took this drug to improve their health it was actually harming their health.[214]

Today statins are a twenty billion dollar a year industry and forty billion people a year are prescribed statins. From what I understand statins, if used, should only be administered on a short term basis. But they are not. I have seen people on statins for 10-15 years and longer. When watching the movie 'Statin Nation', they address that we won't live one day longer taking statins. In fact, they may shorten our life. In the article, The Ugly Side of Statins, adverse side-effects can include kidney failure, liver dysfunction, skin cancer, muscle atrophy, and heart disease.[215]

Yet, Cholesterol fraud is real.

There are several articles that have called attention to the severity of the Cholesterol fraud. "Researchers claim the Cholesterol theory of heart disease is misguided and Cholesterol doesn't cause heart disease." [216]

---

[214] http://www.drugwatch.com/vioxx/recall/

[215] http://www.scirp.org/journal/PaperInformation.aspx?PaperID=34065

[216] http://www.ncbi.nlm.nih.gov/pubmed/18609060

Additionally, it is good to note that statins do play a causative role in ulcerative colitis.[217] Unfortunately, even with all these risks 'Big Pharma' wants to screen children for Cholesterol imbalances as young as nine years of age. A medical rollercoaster ride indeed.

A Bite Size Step:

Are there any fake-food items in your home? Please list them. Can they be replaced with healthy choices?

---

[217] http://pmj.bmj.com/content/78/919/286.full

Some Helpful Tips

Take an active step in your own self-care. For your safety, ask your doctor how many years you need to be on prescribed medications. Toxic Exposures have been proven to have cumulative adverse health effects. *The Reaction?* The body's eliminating systems become impaired. The consequences lead to inflammation, diabetes, obesity, cancer, heart disease and depression.

Health is Interconnected...

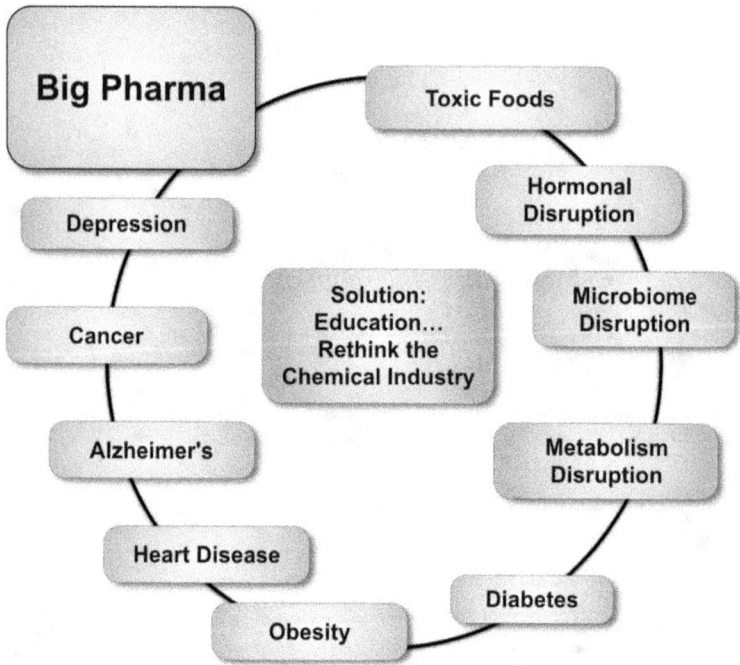

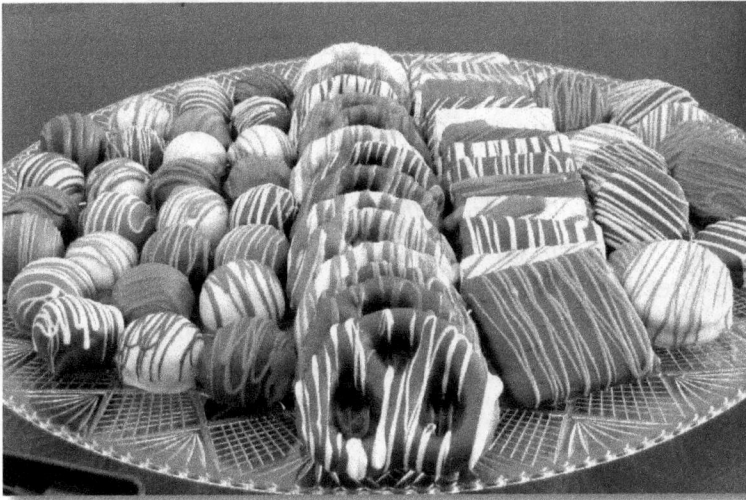

When the body's elimination systems are compromised, pain increases.

Chapter 13

The Elimination / Toxin Connection

Nutrition is the main process of life. Elimination is the second runner-up! Every organ and every cell has a job to process and eliminate. For this to take place, we need to provide all our elimination systems with healthy *Nutrition* and *un-compromised avenues for elimination.*

Every system on the inside is directly affected by what we directly put on it and into it. So we can safely say that when we eat toxins and increase our chances for disease, we can disrupt the normal processes of elimination. Here are thirteen ways the body works overtime to eliminate.

1- **Perspiration:** Sweat is a good thing. Over thirty percent of bodily wastes are eliminated by way of perspiration. What can harm this process? Aluminum and chemicals in Antiperspirants! Antiperspirants mean 'against perspiration.' *The Reaction*: Antiperspirants block sweat glands. Most contain toxic scents. What is most adversely affected are the kidneys and liver. *The Secondary Reaction*: "Antiperspirants can produce radiopaque particles on mammography." [218]

2- **Digestion:** Chemicals and pesticides can interfere with bowel elimination and increase bloating. These can be found in medications, fake foods, sugary drinks, and excitotoxins, just to name a few. A clogged colon can send toxins to the entire body. Eighty percent of Americans are under the influence of these addictive substances. *The Reaction*: A slower and more toxic elimination time. Affected are the immune, metabolic, nervous, circulatory and digestive systems.

---

[218] www.ncbi.nlm.nih.gov/pubmed/24262976

3- **Acidosis:** Every cell is taxed trying to eliminate an acidic environment. According to Dr. Robert Young, a microbiologist and author of '*The pH Miracle*', "the problem with obesity and derivative diseases in this country is that, it's not that we're overweight, it's that we're over acid. An acidic pH can in turn erode and eat into the cell wall. An acidic body cannot effectively maintain high levels of calcium, oxygen or flush out toxins."[219] *The Reaction*: Inflammation. These toxins can remain in our system longer keeping us sick, fat and in pain.[220] "An acidic environment slows down the processing and induction of nutrition going into the cells. The cells communication system and elimination process is then damaged."[221] *The Secondary Reaction*: Acidosis opens the front door to arthritis, IBS, autoimmune disorders, metabolic syndrome and cancer.

When we experience fight or flight symptoms or trauma from social and psychological stressors, inside, these can evoke a similar threat in our immune system, causing the body chemistry to go acidic. How long can this last? It depends on if it's an everyday occurrence. "The experience

---

[219] healthwyze.org/index.php/component/content/article/361-the-relationship-between-body-ph-and-disease-and-other-facts-youre-not-supposed-to-know.html

[220] natural-health-academy.com/natural-health/acidosis/

[221] http://natural-health-academy.com/natural-health/acidosis/

we have today can influence our body composition for the next 80 days." [222]

4- **Pancreatic cancer:** When the pancreas is impaired, the digestive system and kidneys have elimination issues. The digestive system and endocrine system rely on the function of the pancreas. For instance, the pancreas produces enzymes to aid in the digestion process. An impaired pancreas can lead to cancer. "Pancreatic cancer is more common in people with diabetes. *A Negative Process where*: enzymes decrease and allergies and inflammation set in." [223]

5- **Diabetes:** When we have glucose imbalance, we have a kidney impairment. *The Reaction*: The kidneys work harder to eliminate toxins.[224] This in turn affects our gut bacteria and proper bowel elimination. Diabetics can be sensitive to ingesting fluorides. The kidneys handle eliminating fluoride from the body when working optimally. If not, fluoride interrupts urine output,"[225] and alters glucose metabolism.[226]

---

[222] www.theatlantic.com/health/archive/2015/02/what-a-happy-cell-looks-like/385000/?

[223] http://drsircus.com/medicine/sodium-bicarbonate-baking-soda/the-pancreas-bicarbonate-and-diabetes-2

[224] http://www.ncbi.nlm.nih.gov/pubmed/22559853

[225] http://www.ncbi.nlm.nih.gov/pubmed/9456082

[226] http://www.ncbi.nlm.nih.gov/pmc/articles/PMC3657862/

6- **The pituitary gland:** The pituitary gland is an endocrine gland that releases hormones into the bloodstream. Toxic foods, stress and addictions stand in the way of the function of these processes. In fact, a 2005 paper in the journal Brain supported the link between smoking and the risk of developing MS. John McDougall, M.D., cites the British medical journal Lancet in pointing out that a diet filled with dairy products has been closely linked to the development of MS.[227] "The hypothalamus links our nervous system to the endocrine system via the pituitary gland."[228] *The Reaction:* When our organs, nervous system, and glands are toxic they play a role in Alzheimer's disease, Parkinson's disease, and MS.

7- **Prostate cancer:** A toxic prostate is affected by bacteria cells in the gut,[229]sometimes in conjunction with diabetes and poor oral health. A study in the journal, The Prostate, lends further evidence for the "anti-milk" view. "There turned out to be a more than twofold increase in the risk of prostate cancer associated with an increased intake of dairy products."

The Reaction: Sex moves fluid and releases toxins. When fluid is disrupted, men may be put on more than one medication with side-effects that can include sexual

---

[227] The Lancet 1974;2:1061

[228] http://www.ncbi.nlm.nih.gov/pubmed/7009247 see also http://www.ncbi.nlm.nih.gov/pmc/articles/PMC1204764/

[229] http://wp.vcu.edu/masseynews/2013/09/25/bacterial-cells-in-the-gut-found-to-produce-steroid-hormones-that-could-have-implications-for-prostate-and-colon-cancer/

dysfunction. Disfunction in this sense means kidney and colon elimination is impaired.

8- **Liver and Lymph:** Disruption in the liver and lymph may begin with an abundance of Antibiotics, leaving the gut microbiome disrupted. *The Reaction*: The liver has a difficult time with elimination. When bacteria gets into the blood stream, the liver becomes burdened. Excess waste in the intestines can be reabsorbed into the blood and deposited in the liver. The lymphatic drainage area is tied into the colon elimination system as well. If the bowels are plugged, the lymph may have an issue with drainage.[230] Toxins create a stressful body that needs to work harder to release them. Toxins reduce oxygen supply, increasing oxidative stress and premature aging.

9- **Stress:** Most of the time we forget about finding healthy ways to release and eliminate stress. *The Reaction*: Stress can escalate. Not only can stress cause other disorders, but stress also hinders elimination in several body systems. Holding onto stress can increase the risk for cancer, weight gain, constipation, and lower immunity.[231] Stress can increase thyroid disturbances, diabetes, or a heart attack. Stressful events can affect how we breathe and how we hold our breath; hence, liver and lung elimination may be hindered.

---

[230]http://www.gfcn.biz/Better%20Health/Elimination.htm

[231] http://cen.acs.org/articles/90/i34/Brains-Circulatory-System-Clears-Waste.html

10- **The brain:** Imagine going to work every day and exposing yourself regularly to toxic chemicals that are eroding your health. Next time you go into a nail salon, you may want to ask: "Why am I breathing in these chemicals." Toluene is a reproductive toxin and a neurotoxin and enters the body when we breathe. We consume toluene from ground water or have skin contact with it from nail polish. *The Reaction*: Toluene affects the central nervous system, irritates the respiratory system and lymphatic system, and has adverse effects on the kidneys.

11- **Immune System:** Mercury toxicity has been shown to induce auto-immune diseases and is an endocrine disruptor. *The Reaction:* Mercury is excreted through the kidneys and damage can incur leaving the blood filtration system compromised. *The Secondary Reaction*: Damages can also be found in the circulation, endocrine, reproductive and central nervous system.[232] Accumulation of mercury from cosmetics can affect the elimination in the gastrointestinal system. [233]Mercury is an environmental risk factor for cardiovascular disease.[234]

Dr. Rashid Buttar testified before Congress: "the association of mercury to chronic diseases is well documented. The search for the association between mercury and cardiovascular disease and cancer reveals several scientific papers. Anything that depletes and

---

[232]http://www.ncbi.nlm.nih.gov/pmc/articles/PMC3988285/

[233] http://www.ncbi.nlm.nih.gov/pubmed/22070559

[234]http://www.ncbi.nlm.nih.gov/pubmed/18599595

disturbs the immune system will increase one's chances of contracting cancer."[235]

12- **Skin:** Skin is the largest elimination organ of the body and has a relationship to all of our internal organs and body parts. Our skin will eliminate better and smell better when we drink more water.

Consequently, if we eat junk and garbage during the day, we have cellular exhaustion and weakness at night. Reduced nutrition to the epidermis leaves it unable to repair damages and elimination is impaired.[236]

13- **Heart Disease:** Toxins that affect the gut affect the heart. If we experience colon toxicity from a poor diet such as IBS, colitis, and metabolic syndrome, this can be directly linked to poor heart health and heart disease.[237]

The Reaction: Cardiovascular diseases and type 2 diabetes mellitus increases with IBS.[238] In the end, CVD appears to be more common in Irritable Bowel Disorders.[239]

---

[235] http://drsircus.com/medicine/cancer/mercury-and-cancer-research-dental-amalgams

[236] http://blogs.naturalnews.com/lose-weight-sleep/

[237] http://www.ncbi.nlm.nih.gov/pmc/articles/PMC3221110/

[238]http://www.ncbi.nlm.nih.gov/pubmed/24970784

[239] http://www.ncbi.nlm.nih.gov/pubmed/21272803

Each time we choose a favorite toxic food,
suffer from IBS or experience stress,
we can be influencing our health
in several negative directions!

Having suffered colitis and given birth to a colicky baby, I know first-hand that both stem from having poor gut bacteria. Colitis involves the enteric nervous system (*the brain in the gut*) as well as our metabolic and endocrine systems, leaving most elimination systems compromised. Colitis is serious business and most doctors don't talk about how nutrition and proper elimination in all systems play an important role in getting well. I was a long-time user of caffeine and gluten-related products. Both can keep the gut from healing when we suffer from colitis.

A myth is that caffeine stimulates the bowel and therefore we have a healthier elimination system. Caffeine increases an acidic blood level, dehydration, and can be blamed for insomnia. A high caffeine habit depletes the body of B Vitamins, which we need for proper brain function. Caffeine is an endocrine disruptor and contributes to overeating, especially overeating sugar.

A Bite Size Step:
Remember, a sedentary lifestyle makes a sick body & brain.

Some Helpful Tips

Reduce toxicities in your life such as sugar and caffeine and increase movement. All life is movement, so go do it. Exercise is good for the brain, makes us smarter, and helps with all elimination systems.

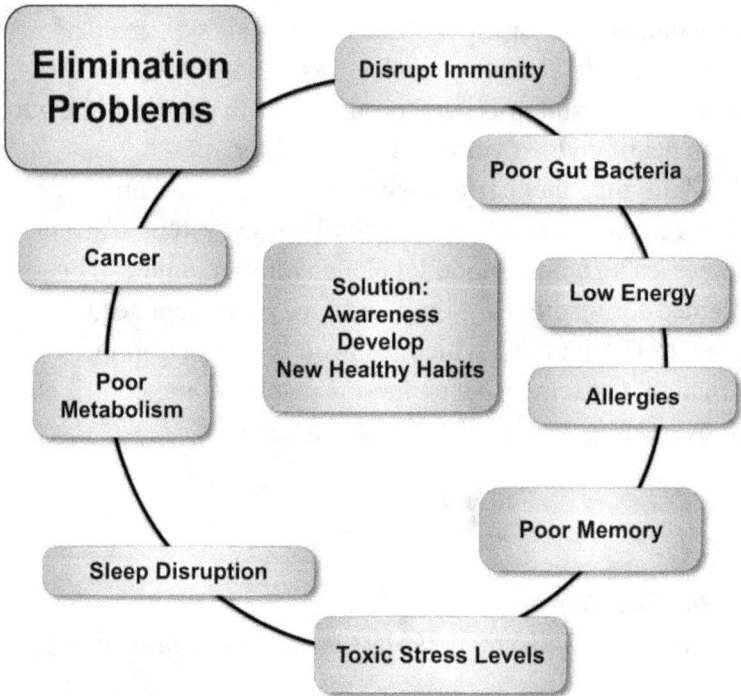

Elimination Problems

Disrupt Immunity

Poor Gut Bacteria

Cancer

Solution:
Awareness
Develop
New Healthy Habits

Low Energy

Poor Metabolism

Allergies

Poor Memory

Sleep Disruption

Toxic Stress Levels

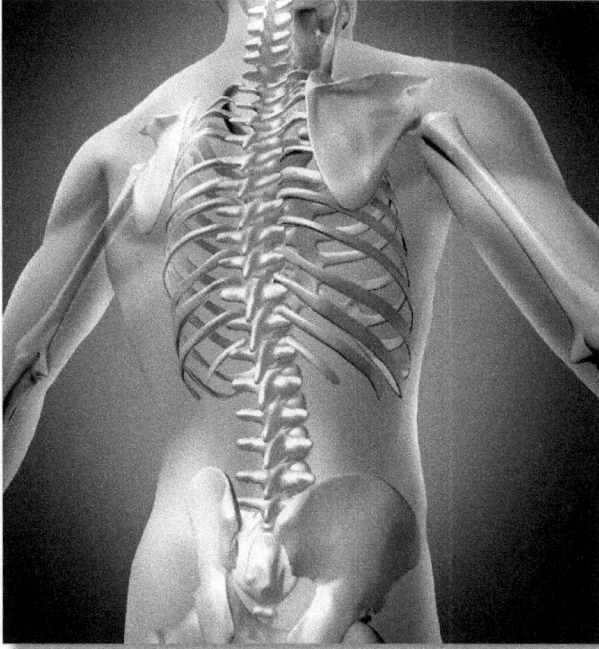

There are things we do on a daily basis,
that can contribute to our discomfort.

Chapter 14

Addressing Inflammation and Pain

Being a certified health coach, numerous clients have asked me how they can reduce their chronic pain and inflammation. What I have discovered is….

Chronic Pain and inflammation is not only linked to poor food choices and toxic exposures, it's linked to Heart Disease, Depression, Obesity, Alzheimer's disease, Autoimmune Disorders, and Cancer.

The body can heal itself when we know the cause.

Meg's Pain

Recently my client Meg asked me how she can relieve her pain from arthritis and RSD (Reflex Sympathetic Dystrophy Syndrome). She also suffered from depression. My research involved months of investigation and here's what I found.

It's safe to say "genes don't cause autoimmune disorders." There are known environmental triggers that initiate the illness. They're called toxic exposures. Besides junk foods, these include varnishes and glues (organic solvents), toxic paints, and dry cleaning solvents.[240]

Meg's daily dietary choices included breads, crackers, GMO cheesy pizzas (a high gluten diet), alcohol, diet drinks, processed meats, french fries and tons of sugar at each meal and/or snack. Interestingly, gluten sensitivity can

---

[240] http://www.ncbi.nlm.nih.gov/pmc/articles/PMC3526640/

keep us in a depressive state just like sugar and includes fatigue and musculoskeletal pains.[241] In fact, an abundance of sugar and gluten products disrupt hormones, increase fat, inflammation and insulin resistance.[242]

There was exposure to several chemicals and toxins in her home as well as in the salon and dry cleaners she frequented once a week. Money wasn't an issue, yet she never considered purchasing organic meats, fruits or veggies. She said her kids wouldn't eat them. Everyday habits included fast foods, cereals with milk, caffeine with powdered creamers, GMO eggs with white toast, boxed and canned foods, french fries with trans-fats and processed-meats such as bacon and pepperoni on her pizza. Processed meat can be linked to cancer.[243] All of her dietary habits can cause inflammation in the mind and body.

Mounting evidence shows inflammation, PAIN and fatty adipose tissue plays a causative role in autoimmune disorders. Adiposity (fat tissue) can be a risk factor for inflammation, heart disease, diabetes, and cancer. It adds to poor brain health, poor gut bacteria, to poor renal function.[244] A toxic lifestyle has lead to Meg's chronic pain and inflammation.

Meg was obese from poor food choices, an abundance of medications, and chemical exposures. As found in Chapter 7, obesity opens the door for estrogen

---

[241]https://sites.google.com/site/jccglutenfree/depression,anxiety,panic

[242] http://www.ncbi.nlm.nih.gov/pubmed/23253599

[243] http://www.livescience.com/52651-red-meat-cancer-warning-explained.html

[244]http://www.researchgate.net/publication/276157277_Urinary_metabolic_signatures_of_human_adiposity

dominance.[245] My research included studies that linked toxic chemical exposures to the rise of chronic diseases.[246]

"C-reactive protein is a protein found in the blood, the levels of which rise in reaction to inflammation."[247] The inflammation signaled by (CRP) is influenced by exposure to environmental toxins and diet, particularly one that contains a lot of refined, processed and sugary foods. CRP is an inflammation marker that plays a key role in depression.[248]

Obesity can make inflammation worse and antidepressants can play a causative role in obesity. Meg was addicted to antidepressants.

Meg drank large amounts of wine every night. Alcohol use and a high sugar diet is never recommended for nerve damage and can worsen chronic pain and inflammation. We can only be neglectful for so long before the body's elimination system is in jeopardy.

RSD can affect the immune system in the brain, the skin and the gut. RSD can be linked to circulation

---

[245]http://www.scientificamerican.com/article/antibiotics-linked-weight-gain-mice/

[246] http://www.post-gazette.com/news/nation/2010/01/22/stricter-rules-urged-on-toxic-chemicals/201001220218

[247]https://en.wikipedia.org/wiki/Acute-phase_protein Wikipedia®

[248]http://archpsyc.jamanetwork.com/article.aspx?articleid=1485898 see also http://media.jamanetwork.com/news-item/elevated-levels-of-c-reactive-protein-appear-associated-with-psychological-distress-depression/

dysfunction because of the constriction of the blood vessels.[249]

When working properly, the brain's circulatory system clears waste. When not, toxic exposures can buildup and pave the way toward Alzheimer's Disease.[250] When Meg realized the path she was taking was only making her feel worse, she listened.

Some Helpful Tips

Non steroidal anti-inflammatory medication (NSAID's) can actually increase leaky gut, which in turn increases inflammation. PAIN is a warning sign/a symptom. Chronic pain decreases brain function. Pain can be related to dehydration or we may be chemically toxic. As a society, we need to ask ourselves: "how is continuing a toxic lifestyle going to ease our pain?" It won't. The good news…When neglect stops, healing happens!

---

[249]http://www.rsdcanada.org/parc/english/RSD-CRPS/whatis.html

[250] .http://cen.acs.org/articles/90/i34/Brains-Circulatory-System-Clears-Waste.html

My Friend is Tox-Sick

Did you ever find yourself not feeling well, but didn't know what to do? My good friend, Jane, drove herself to the hospital last year, because after taking all of her prescribed medications with additional NSAID's, she still was experiencing excruciating headaches, dizziness, joint pain and a sick stomach. She brags about how exceptional her insurance company is that she was able to receive all the top notch tests. She said: "We take it all for granted, but it's pretty amazing that there is a place we can go to take care of emergencies and get the right medication. They can tell me in 10 minutes if I have a brain tumor or not. And with the right Medicare plan it cost zero even to go to the Mayo Clinic." Jane's test included MRI's, CAT scans, blood analysis and the Ultrasound of her Aortic Valve. Surprisingly enough, nothing was found.

I'm familiar with her habits, so I asked, "When was the last time you had a drink of water?" She barked "I just finished a diet cola and had three cups of coffee today." My inquiry continued with: "Is your medication still the same?" "Not really", she said, "I added sleeping pills and an acid reflux medication while my statin medication remains the same." In the same breath, she claimed they had scheduled her for more tests on Tuesday.

Her headache returned. Aspartame has a strong mall-effect on the functioning of the brain. So in my pursuit to be helpful, I suggested she cease diet colas for a few days and to include more water. She didn't agree. I continued with: "do you know any of the side-effects from your medications?" She said "her doctors know all about what her needs are." OMG. Did I really hear that? I thought— Wow, how can I encourage one tiny "bite size step" with such a closed mind?

If we ask: "Can the body heal itself?" The answer is YES. However, if we don't have that belief system in place, who do we think does the healing? Science?

The final word from those doctor visits and the Mayo clinic, all tests came back negative. No brain tumor - yet!

Everything we do involves energy. We get energy from the frequency of our food source. If we eat 'toxic food', we get toxic energy. Living on processed foods, day in and day out, can leave us sick and lethargic because toxic frequency doesn't feed our cells. It leaves us with a toxic mind and body.

The way to influence anything is not to control circumstances but to learn how to control our thoughts. Foods and thoughts are connected. You may have heard the energy of your food becomes your mind. One teacher, I enjoyed learning from at the Institute for Integrative Nutrition® was David Wolfe. David Wolfe said: "You can't drink soda pop and expect to have noble thoughts." And he was right.[251]

A Bite Size Step:
Ask yourself: What influences your symptoms? Can you release your toxic load to help relieve your pain. And remember, never give up!

---

[251] http://EzineArticles.com/7176735

Some Helpful Tips

Want to get out of pain and bring the joy back into your life? You can begin by introducing 5 organic foods a week into your diet.

Cinnamon has been found to be good for pain.[252]

Using fresh ginger root and making an appointment for ice massage therapy for inflammation and pain relief is safe and easy to implement.

When we feel good all the time,
we want to live a full and joyful life. If we don't,
moods, discomfort, and pain get in the way of life.

---

[252] http://www.ncbi.nlm.nih.gov/pmc/articles/PMC4437117/

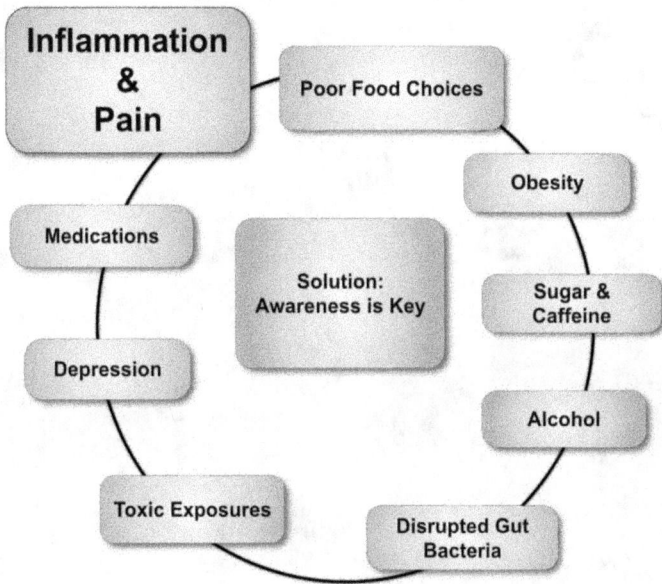

Inflammation & Pain
Poor Food Choices
Obesity
Sugar & Caffeine
Alcohol
Disrupted Gut Bacteria
Toxic Exposures
Depression
Medications
Solution: Awareness is Key

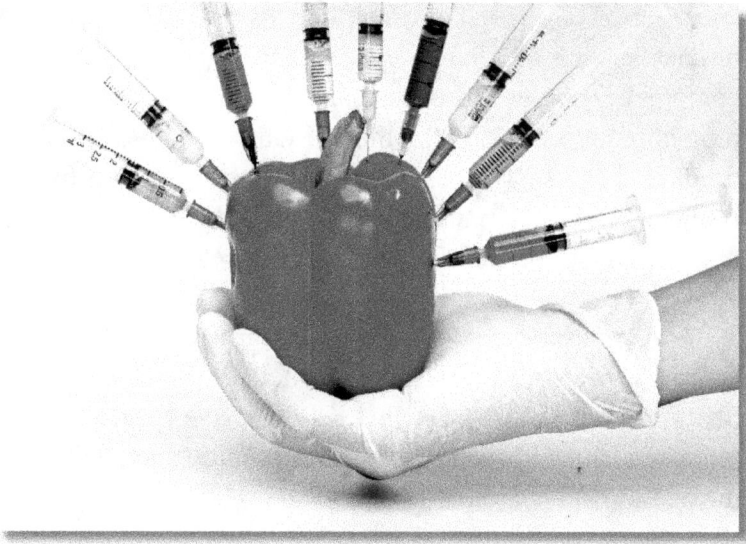

How do we keep from being deceived by the latest, expertly, scientific deceptive propaganda techniques?

Chapter 15

Unsafe Science

With so much misinformation floating around how do we choose who and what to believe? Who can we trust for the latest accurate verified information? And what is junk, fake or unsafe science? There are more than 300,000 scientific conferences and events each year. Many are funded by the drug corporations. In 2003, the UK Guardian revealed that drug companies pay ghostwriters to write nearly half of the research articles. These can appear in medical journals to promote prescription drugs.[253]

Fake science was created so the pharmaceutical companies can get doctors to push their drugs.[254] As told by Shayrl Attkisson on TEDx TALK: "We have special interest designed to manipulate your opinion about taking medications."[255]

Confusing Science believes: "It could be possible to curb or even reverse the epidemic of obesity by changing aspects of the external environment. People tend to lose weight when entering college, moving or getting a divorce."[256] They don't mention changing our internal environment with real whole foods will be more sustainable. Losing weight under stressful events can keep our mind and body sick, tired and depressed.

---

[253] http://www.theguardian.com/society/2003/dec/07/health.businessofresearch

[254]http://www.npr.org/sections/health-shots/2013/10/03/228859954/some-online-journals-will-publish-fake-science-for-a-fee

[255] https://youtu.be/-bYAQ-ZZtEU

[256] http://www.ncbi.nlm.nih.gov/pubmed/16263145

Deceptive Science: It has been noted that doctors may prescribe chemotherapy even if they know we may not need it. [257] We may find financial incentives and profits takes higher precedence than human life. The Hippocratic Oath has been violated. "First do no harm" (I will neither give a deadly drug to anybody that ask for it).[258]

More Deceptive Science: Imagine you have to sign a waiver from a hospital that's about to perform surgery on you saying: "I accept the greater risk of complications and even death." If we think this is a rare occurrence, think again.[259]

A Bite Size Step:
Become aware of waivers you may be asked to sign in a doctors office or a school program.

---

[257] http://www.marketplace.org/topics/life/study-financial-incentive-pushes-doctors-prescribe-chemo

[258] http://guides.library.jhu.edu/c.php?g=202502&p=1335752

[259] http://www.usnews.com/opinion/blogs/policy-dose/2015/06/03/low-volume-hospitals-create-big-risks-for-surgery-patients

A False High

When I teach in high schools, I hear teenagers say, "How do I get more energy?" "I'd like to have more energy to be able to study and play." Or, "it seems I spend my week recovering from the weekend before."

These kids visit the grocers hoping to find a new energy booster drink, and there's plenty to choose from!

The great food hoax doesn't advise us that water is paramount for energy. We think we're going to find energy in a caffeine and sugary store bought bottle. And, we're willing to pay the price. We're not thinking - 'is this going to help me sustain a long healthy life?' We don't care. We made an unconscious decision to say YES to it. It's happening daily. We're duped into chemically created drink-stuff, which isn't safe to drink. It's a crime in and of itself that puts our children at risk for serious illnesses.[260]

Alternative practitioners say there are no safety tests performed on these experimental drinks. While researchers with published findings say steer clear of these energy drinks until further notice.[261]

It's human nature to crave energy. But reaching for junk food, alcohol, medications or other chemicals to give us energy is never the answer. *The Reaction:* We've become so sick we are tox-sick. The irony is more energy is lost because of poor eating and drinking habits. We've depressed our energy system (mitochondria) and increased oxidative stress in the body. **M**itochondria are power

---

[260]http://www.ncbi.nlm.nih.gov/pmc/articles/PMC3065144/

[261] http://med.miami.edu/news/um-pediatric-researchers-publish-findings-on-energy-drinks

bundles that give our organs energy.[262] With disruptive Mitochondria, we increased our risk for illness. These illnesses include but are not limited to cancer, heart disorders and diabetes. Mitochondrial dysfunction and oxidative stress are associated with abnormal brain function and mood disorders, such as depression. [263] All these can lead us down the road to Alzheimer's disease.[264]

---

[262]http://www.askdrray.com/preserving-our-energy/

[263]http://www.ncbi.nlm.nih.gov/pmc/articles/PMC3640606/

[264] http://www.ncbi.nlm.nih.gov/pubmed/15377876

What is unsafe about Science?
What is promoted as safe, is not.

Unsafe science...

According to journals.plos.org, genes may pass from food to human blood and cause problems in our digestive tract.[265] Unsafe science can be negatively altering our cells[266] with the consequences of increasing obesity, diabetes, and even death, while our own government has given certain food giants immunity from lawsuits.[267]

***

According to the organization proton.org, [268]the following *unsafe* reactions were found in the five medications listed below.

1-A painkiller medication Duract. *The reactions* - liver damage, liver transplants and death.

2-A diabetic medication Rezulin. *The reactions* - liver failure and death.

---

[265] http://journals.plos.org/plosone/article?id=10.1371/journal.pone.0069805

[266] http://www.ncbi.nlm.nih.gov/pmc/articles/PMC3955666/

[267] http://www.globalresearch.ca/monsanto-protection-act-signed-by-obama-gmo-bill-written-by-monsanto-signed-into-law/5329388

[268] http://prescriptiondrugs.procon.org/view.resource.php?resourceID=005528

3-An irritable bowel medication Lotronex. *The reactions* - causes inflammation and injury in the small intestine.

4-An irritable bowel medication Zelnorm. *The reactions* - increased risk for heart attack and stroke.

5-An appetite suppressant Meridia. *The Reaction -* Increased cardiovascular illness.

***

In the early 1900's trans-fats were hailed as excellent for heart health. We believed the advertising that said: "everything cooked better in Crisco."[269] It was 1913 when reports of problems began to appear—problems like increased heart disease, increased cancer, growth problems, learning disorders and infertility while P&G worked behind the scenes to cover them up.[270]

Margarine is still being promoted as healthy.[271] And just when we thought removing trans-fats by 2016 would

---

[269]http://www.realfoodhouston.com/2013/05/20/crisco-how-marketing-trumped-nutrition/

[270] http://wp.me/p1otL6-eE

[271] http://www.hsph.harvard.edu/nutritionsource/what-should-you-eat/fats-and-cholesterol/

be a giant step in the right direction, trans-fats are just being re-labeled.[272]

***

The pasteurization process contributes to big profits and toxins.[273] Television commercials and grade schools push the idea that 'milk is a health food.' Don't be fooled with myths and misinformation about the quality of your milk.[274] "The initiation phase of cancer from bovine milk products can begin early in a child's life."[249]

***

Health Claims on food packaging can be extremely manipulatory and appeal to our emotions. In the U.S. more people say they want to be more health conscious than ever. Food manufacturers are well aware of this and have found ways to market even to the health conscious by adding misleading labels and misleading marketing claims. These are used to trick people into thinking that they're making the right choice for themselves and their family.[275]

---

[272] http://civileats.com/2015/06/19/4-things-you-should-know-about-fdas-ban-on-trans-fats/

[273] https://foodfreedom.wordpress.com/2009/11/24/pasteurization-pulling-the-plug-on-scientific-fallacies-undergirding-our-industrial-food-and-drug-culture/

[274] http://www.nutritionandmetabolism.com/content/9/1/74 see also http://saveourbones.com/osteoporosis-milk-myth/

[275] http://www.eatdrinkpolitics.com/wp-content/uploads/SimonWhitewashedDairyReport.pdf

***

A Chemo bath is an invasive "treatment" with many side-effects. Doctors remove several organs just in case these organs may be cancerous before administering 107-degree chemo inside the stomach/colon.[276] I had a client that opted to have this done. He passed away while recovering. Surgery is not curative or part of cancer control, if you are not addressing the cause.

No studies establish efficacy for chemo baths. [277] Unfortunately, for the first time, you may be hearing that treatments for Cancer is not science- based.[278]

***

What else leads to cancer? Smoking. According to their own website,[279] Pfizer describes the side-effects from the drug Chantix. These side-effects include seizures, heart problems, thoughts of suicide, trouble breathing, and death. This drug is used to help people to stop smoking.[280]

---

[276] http://www.dailymail.co.uk/health/article-2130648/Amazing-chemo-bath-saves-cancer-patients-doctors-wrote-off.html

[277] http://nursing.onclive.com/publications/oncology-nurse/2011/december-2011/Chemo-Controversy-An-Inside-Look-at-Hot-Chemotherapy-Bath

[278]http://thetruthaboutcancer.com/truth-behind-science-based-medicine/

[279] http://labeling.pfizer.com/ShowLabeling.aspx?id=557

As a nation, we failed to act on a body of evidence to eliminate exposure to carcinogens.

Unsafe Exposures

Dioxins are chemicals in the environment and found in meat and dairy products. These are endocrine disruptors that can cause hyperactivity, lowered testosterone levels, cancer and more.[281] Several epidemiological studies have indicated a relationship between dairy consumption and breast cancer risk in **pre-menopausal women.**[282] Additionally, findings show that diets high in meat may cause cancer.[283]

PCBs are man-made chemicals and are endocrine disruptors. They are in the air, soil, and water supply. They have been found to cause cancer.[284]

---

[281] http://www.ncbi.nlm.nih.gov/pmc/articles/PMC1241417/pdf/ehp0111-000389.pdf

[282] http://www.breastcancerfund.org/clear-science/radiation-chemicals-and-breast-cancer/bovine-growth-hormone.html

[283] http://www.mdpi.com/2072-6643/6/1/163/htm

[284] http://www.ncbi.nlm.nih.gov/pubmed/11914190

Where is Safety Missing?

1. Fluoride Ingestion Isn't Safe

Imagine drugging children for years with fluoridation and when we refuse we are labeled crazy. In 1979 that's what happened to me. In the U.S., it is extremely difficult to opt out of water fluoridation, fluoride vitamins, and the fluoride dominated American Dental Association. As found in Chapter 13, Fluoride is an excitotoxin, meaning it disrupts brain cells. It is understood that children exposed to fluoride have lower IQ levels.[285]

2. Vaccines Aren't Safe

My son was not sick before his first vaccine back in the late 70's. On that fateful day of his first MMR (measles, mumps, rubella vaccination), he screamed a high pitch scream and couldn't be consoled. A fever started and escalated to 104 degrees. Within a half-hour he convulsed (went into a seizure) in my arms, turned white and then blue. For a minute, all sound stopped. I was alone and thought he was dead.

I dialed 911 with my pinky finger. We were rushed to the hospital emergency room where they wanted permission to give him a spinal tap. I declined. Why? There were two reasons:

First, I was asked to sign a waiver if they accidentally caused injury to the blood vessels surrounding my son's spine.

---

[285]http://www.hsph.harvard.edu/news/features/fluoride-childrens-health-grandjean-choi/

Second, I could so clearly see the set of circumstances involving vaccinations. I thought, "why couldn't the doctors?"

I recalled Connie Chung on CBS bringing up the possibility of 'questioning your doctor' about the risk of vaccinations. I did. My doctor told me the risk was ONE in one million.[286] This was not the truth. Imagine a new mother (me) traumatized by almost losing her son.

This was my first tox-sick wake-up call!

I did a little research for you and here's what I found. There's junk and fake science informing us about vaccine safety, while profits are mostly behind vaccine science. Here are a few on how vaccines harm.[287] Here is selling junk science.[288] And here are "profits not science" that motivate vaccines mandates.[289] My son's immune system was clearly in danger after his first vaccine because of several toxins entering his tiny body at once.

----

[286] http://blogs.naturalnews.com/viruses-really-cut-short-vaccines/

[287] http://www.nvic.org/vaccines-and-diseases/Vaccinations--Know-the-risks-and-failures-.aspx see also https://vaccineimpact.com/2014/dr-andrew-moulden-every-vaccine-produces-harm/

[288] http://www.anh-usa.org/selling-junk-science/

[289] https://www.wellbeingjournal.com/profits-not-science-motivate-vaccine-mandates/

3. Cutting The Fat Isn't Safe

First they get us fat. Then they cut it off! Bariatric Surgery for diabetes and obesity is not the answer for fat loss, obesity or diabetes. For a surgery this invasive one must look at the complications that may include death, leaking stomach acid, depression, heart attack, bleeding, blood clots and nutritional deficiencies. (This surgery adds in a lifetime of medications and deletes certain foods we can no longer digest.) Type 2 diabetes can lead to cancer.[290] Can cutting the fat prevent that? I think not.

Attaining the ideal weight can be difficult without the ideal mindset. Weight loss needn't be about dieting, pills or bariatric surgery that can lead to death.[291] It's about decision making and a powerful mindset to follow through.

4. ADD is More Than Just Attention Deficit

Our children are put on dangerous life threatening medications for ADD that may cause several side-effects, while many parents seem to think they don't have a choice in the matter.[292] Have you ever felt like you didn't have a choice about your child's health? I did. The school system insisted I put my child on Ritalin for a language disorder. I opted out and opted into homeschooling. I enrolled in homeschool groups, attended conferences with other homeschool moms and bought tons of books. I also hired several tutors. It wasn't easy but well worth it.

---

[290] http://www.ncbi.nlm.nih.gov/pubmed/20309918

[291] http://www.ncbi.nlm.nih.gov/pubmed/20960546 see also
http://care.diabetesjournals.org/content/28/2/472.full

[292] http://www.healthfreedoms.org/toddlers-dosed-with-speed-how-big-pharma-hooks-americas-kids-on-dangerous-meds/

Some Helpful Tips

There are several toxins children can be exposed to on a regular basis. In fact, children can be born toxic.

Food can be our first line of defense for ADD. A child's brain can be disrupted by pesticides[293] as well as food allergies. Foods that a child can be sensitive to are sugar, dairy, soy, caffeine, wheat, and corn. A sensitivity to wheat can be a result of insecticides and unwanted hormones sprayed prior to germination.

Medications such as amphetamines given for ADD can cause mitochondrial dysfunction and increase oxidative stress.[294]

Given that most people believe they are a victim of their genes, helpless to starve off some of the most dreaded diseases, they are not. We aren't helpless at all. In fact, the power is largely in our own hands. It's called mindset.[295]

---

[293] http://www.ncbi.nlm.nih.gov/pubmed/18032333

[294] http://www.ncbi.nlm.nih.gov/pubmed/11198300

[295] http://www.medicalnewstoday.com/releases/197733.php

Finding Clarity in an Insane World

"The psych drug market is in the range of 40 billion dollars a year. Every day 850 adults and 250 children are added to the disability criteria for mental health reasons." It's time to take our health back in mind and body. Big Pharma has not proven to cure the depression crisis.[296]

Unfortunately more often than not we have corporations trying to Deceive America. According to healthfreedoms.org "Glaxo Smith Kline" must pay out $3 billion for the fraudulent sale and marketing of drugs including the popular antidepressant Wellbutrin." [297] Taking our health back requires us to be informed and become empowered in mind and body health.

A Bite Size Step:
Give yourself permission to breathe. Explore your beliefs.
Empower yourself. When you do, the body has a chance to
heal itself!

---

[296] http://www.healthfreedoms.org/big-pharma-cant-cure-the-mental-illness-crisis/

[297] http://www.healthfreedoms.org/how-big-pharma-and-dr-drew-made-a-fortune-deceiving-america/

Some Helpful Tips

Why wait until you are sick, tired and obese before you consider wellness? Begin building your immunity now with foods that can feed your cells. It's the immune system that heals the body.

Don't be afraid to question your doctor about the side-effects of your medication. Ask: "Is managing my disease with pills that eventually add to the progression of my disease and eventual death, unsafe science?"

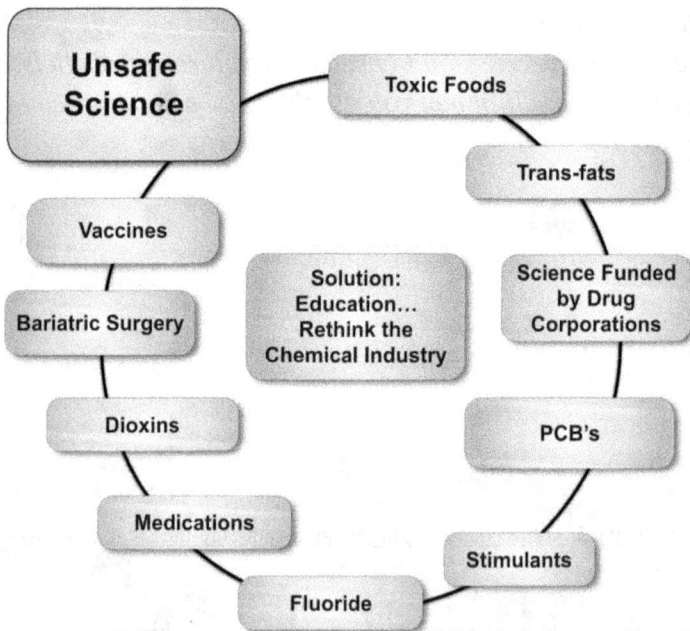

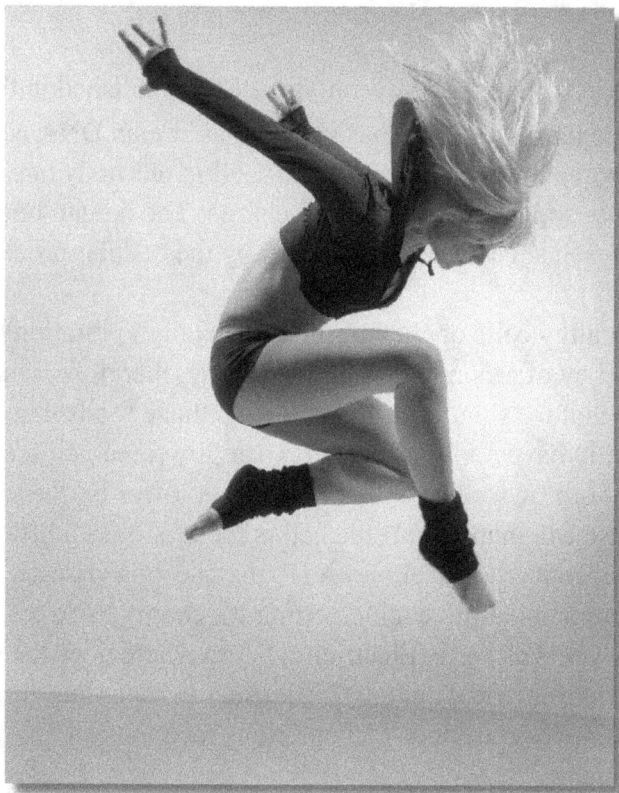

The Ancient Master of Taoism Lao Tzu teaches:
"The journey of 1,000 miles,
begins with one step."

Chapter 16

The Body is Electric!

Bio-electricity involves the cell membrane.

Research from the University of Basel, published in the science journal Nature, has shown that human DNA can transport electrical current. Every cell in our body has a positive and negative electrical charge. The human body vibrates in several patterns caused by the cellular process we call life.

Healthy cells operate optimally at a high vibration frequency of around 60 to 80 megahertz, therefore it makes sense that we should ideally consume those foods that naturally have a vibration energy (or 'life force') closest to that of our own cells. Why? Because at lower frequencies dis-ease can manifest. If the cell is thought of as a little red engine, converting fuel into ATP, the question arises: "Where is this little engine getting it's energy to do it's job?" The Answer is Electricity! "And where does the cell store this electrical charge?" The Answer is in the cell membrane. Both foods and emotions feed the cell membrane.

If more than seventy-five percent of all cancers are preventable, then why is cancer still harming 1 in 3? Cancer manifests at lower frequencies.

We are more than just a body. We have feelings, we are emotional, we are spiritual, we have minds – we are mental beings. The mind is an energetic field, which can experience 'wear and tear issues'. Science proves that mind, body, spirit and emotions constantly interact and when sickness is in any one of those areas, the other is affected.[298]

Robert O. Becker, M.D., the author of the book: *The Body Electric* validates that the human body has an electrical frequency and that much about a person's health can be determined by it.

Plus...

Nikola Tesla said: " ...if you could eliminate certain outside frequencies that interfered in our bodies, we would have greater resistance toward disease. Beyond a doubt, certain frequencies can prevent the development of disease and other frequencies would destroy diseases."

Wear and Tear Issues

As the body breaks down, inflammation from toxic exposures depletes our energy.

"The Pineal Gland is a magneto-sensitive organ and what that means is, it's sensitive to electromagnetic fields (EMF)."[299] What disrupts this gland includes Wi-Fi, hairdryers, fluoride, stress, diet drinks, computer monitors, microwave ovens to high voltage lines and more. "Electromagnetic fields affect brain waves and suppress the activity of the Pineal Gland and reduce melatonin

---

[298]http://www.ncbi.nlm.nih.gov/pmc/articles/PMC1142191/ see also (http://www.iempowerself.com/52_energy_law_of_attraction.html

[299]Demaine C., Semm P. 1985. The avian pineal gland as an independent magnetic sensor. Neurosci. Lett. 62, 119–122

production"[300] resulting in insomnia.[301] Wi-Fi brings with it wear and tear.

Toxic energy. Toxic emotions such as 'anger' drains our energy as does stress and negative thoughts. [302]When we are feeling emotional, our whole being can take on that energy. Toxic relationships can deplete our vibrational frequencies, depleting our energy levels in our body and mind. Even after a traumatic event is over and forgotten that energy can still be trapped inside, disrupting the flow and distorting the tissues around it. Every one of us has years of emotions trapped in stored cellular energy. Trapped emotions can be toxic to the immune system and elimination system. *The Reaction:* Disrupted immunity. This is where emotions can truly hurt us if we let them fester.

According to Fritz Frederick Smith, "the body compensates for energetic or vibratory loss." "When there is energetic deficiency, the body attempts to limit further loss by reducing its function." A deficiency can lead us down the road to ill health and many disorders that have an interrelationship with low frequency. Low frequency includes neuropathy, depression, obesity, diabetes, heart disease, and cancer.

Illnesses begin and multiply first with lost electrical integrity. This is the consequence of a toxic mind and a

---

[300]http://www.hindawi.com/journals/bmri/2014/169459/

[301]http://www.patient.co.uk/doctor/pineal-gland-and-circadian-rhythms

[302]http://www.askdrray.com/preserving-our-energy/

toxic body. When we pollute our inner environment, it strips our electrical charges.

What about salt?

Over the past few decades, the medical industry put sodium on the bad list and got people to restrict or even cut out salt in their diet. As humans we have a salt history. Our body is an amazing balance of over 50+ trillion cells. In addition to our cells we have over 50 + trillion bacteria in our gut. This creates a balance of both biochemistry and bio-electricity. For thousands of years, sodium has been looked at as one of the fundamental components of health.

When we cut sodium but still eat junk foods, a problem arises. What happens next is our systems can go into emergency mode, holding on to every drop of water it can find. Thus swelling!

Most toxic salts in our diet are found in fast food restaurants, pastry shops, store bought roasted nuts, chips, dips, salsa, cereals, crackers, breads, canned foods, and more. These salts can contain chlorine. The side-effects from these alone can retain fluid in the body and create a puffy look all over. Unfortunately these can also cause unwanted weight gain, digestive issues, and can leach magnesium from our body.

Some Helpful Tips

Food is energy and information. Nutritious foods from Mother Nature's Table feed our mind and body. If we eat junk, energy is lost.

Having a 'Healthy Metabolism' is all about energy. Eating for health involves supporting all of the electrical systems in the body with extremely high-quality nutrients. There is energy and healing powers in colors in everything we do in our life. The colors we choose in our foods is no exception. Invite color onto your plate at your next meal. Make it Art! Brighten up your palettes. Feel the love. Choose a plate of colorful organic vegetables, fruits, soups, and salads. With this powerful 'language of color,' you can discover how to use it to enhance your well-being, prevent illnesses and fill your mind and body with energy.

By now we have become aware that dis-ease can begin with the decline of electrical integrity within the body. Because 80% of our immune system is in our gut, it's important to become aware of toxic foods and exposures that can negatively impact this bioelectrical component of optimal health.

Like any other training we do for our body (football or soccer) to stay physically fit we also have to include the mind muscle. And for us to stay physically fit in all areas, we need to practice often. With time we are capable of changing our path, our results and reinventing our very being.

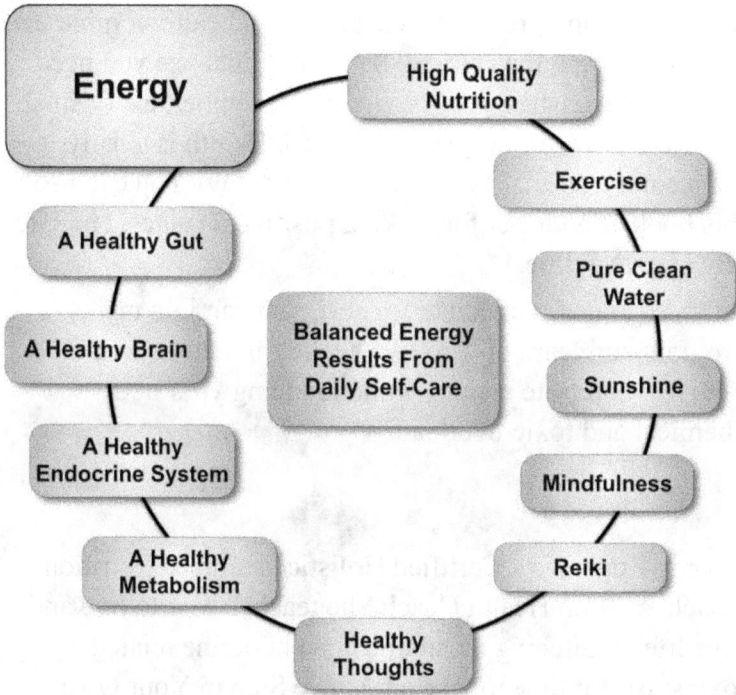

Energy

High Quality Nutrition

Exercise

A Healthy Gut

Pure Clean Water

Balanced Energy Results From Daily Self-Care

A Healthy Brain

Sunshine

A Healthy Endocrine System

Mindfulness

A Healthy Metabolism

Reiki

Healthy Thoughts

It's human nature to want to move away from illness and into feeling great! Make a plan for a healthier mind and body by getting the support, help, and guidance you need from my 'toxic-free you' program. Remember, every small change starts with just a step forward. Health is a daily choice not a special event. Reclaim it today! You can use this book as a toolkit for making positive changes, one bite size step at a time.

If you need immediate support, you can join my program and learn how to live healthy in a toxic world.[303] See, feel and taste results, while reducing your body's chemical and toxic overload.

Connie Rogers is a Certified Holistic Health & Nutrition Coach & Brain Health Coach She teaches how to live and love life by ditching metabolic and endocrine related toxins. Isn't it time to take an Active Step in Your Own Healing?

---

[303] https://bitesizepieces.lpages.co/steps-to-get-toxins-out/

Testimonials:

"Connie shared some great detox information a few years ago that helped reduce a goiter in my thyroid gland and helped me avoid surgery for thyroid removal and years of medication to follow... Thanks Connie"

S. Meade, July, 2015

"I was having a great deal of trouble and pain in my SI joints and low back while on vacation. Connie noticed this and offered a Reiki Session which I readily accepted. I have only heard of Reiki, but have no knowledge of it. The session was very relaxing. My last sensation before going into a dream state was that of heat emanating from her hands when placed in proximity to me. The session lasted about an hour. The major result that I noticed was an increase in general energy over the next 4-5 days and an improved mental attitude."
Regards,

Dr. Clark, Dentist - May, 2014

"I just really appreciate so much about who you are, what you do, and how you do it. Rarely do I meet someone as knowledgeable, responsible, thorough, and communicative as I've seen you to be. And I WISH that more people were like you."

T. Bergenn, 2014

_____

"Over the years I have really never given much thought about what I was eating. For the past three years I was noticing my energy levels declining. In the past six months my health had totally gone down hill to the point that I was literally coughing and choking for air until I would actually pass out. My doctor finally admitted me into the hospital where I spent the next three weeks.

After being in the hospital for three weeks the doctors put me on a medication that was going to cost me between $4500 to $6000 a month. I couldn't afford this. My Cholesterol and blood pressure was high. But, on top of that I was told by my doctor that I had only about three to four months to live, because of cancer. I was just devastated by what they had to say.

They had put me on a drug called Octreotide / Sandostatin. This drug made me feel so bad, and was so expensive ,that I just couldn't make myself live the rest of my life using it. This is when I confided in a friend and I was telling him what was going on with my health. He then introduced me to Connie, who is now my health coach. When I found Connie, I was totally committed to do what I had to in order to feel better and life. I wanted to see my grandkids grow up. My intention was to prove the doctors wrong. I started working with Connie using her program to reduce toxins. I feel so much better now than I have felt in three years.

I totally changed my eating habits and stop eating my daily habits of refined sugars, processed dairy, and gluten products. I juice three times a day and eat a lot of healthy vegetables and wild salmon. My stomach feels a lot better. I have no more headaches or depression. My blood pressure is now normal after two years of being on high blood pressure medication. I don't take any more pain medications today. My coughing is gone. My acid reflux is gone. My knees hurt for ten years and now they no longer hurt like they did before. I have lost 37 pounds! Thank you Connie. You have really helped me understand the importance of new habits."
"Now Off Multiple Meds and Feeling Better Each Day!"

Doug L., November, 2013

"Connie is the top's in her field!! You are treated like royalty, very personable and caring."

Wil, May 26, 2011

_____

"My coaching program with Connie has proven invaluable. She offered me a program that was target specific to my individual needs. I have found ways to relieve my pain from fibromyalgia. I feel better, have more energy, weigh less and my back pain has decreased 80%. She was very knowledgeable and patient while supporting me through many changes. She encourages her clients to be all that they can be and is committed to you and your results. I appreciate her listening skills, energy and expertise. Knowing that she allowed a safe space for me to grow and make changes at my own pace, I would recommend her to all my friends. I feel very thankful that she has come into my life."

Michelle Z., Nevada 12/ 2012

_____

"We have known Connie for years now and highly recommend her as a reliable, creative, fun, caring individual. We have observed her consistently displaying an outstanding work and home ethic. She is very well versed in holistic health. We cannot recommend Connie more highly for any endeavor that would engage her special skill set – weight loss, healthy meal preparations and holistic health coaching."

Heidi M., July 2012

_____

To contact the author, visit www.bitesizepieces.net
ISBN 978-0692566066
Printed in the United States of America

Final Thoughts:

Decades of work created my passion to seek out the truth about health. I hope this becomes a "go to work book", when you have concerns or questions about personal health issues.

When in doubt investigate for yourself. Knowledge is power when applied. The greater our foundation of knowledge, the more we take back our power to be in charge of our health.

All footnotes are working at time of publication.

For better health, I invite you to join me here: **https:// bitesizepieces.lpages.co/steps-to-get-toxins-out/**

Thank you so much and here's to your health!

Connie Rogers

www.ingramcontent.com/pod-product-compliance
Lightning Source LLC
Chambersburg PA
CBHW062223270326
41930CB00009B/1849